Overview on Echinococcosis

Edited by Fethi Derbel and Meriem Braiki

Published in London, United Kingdom

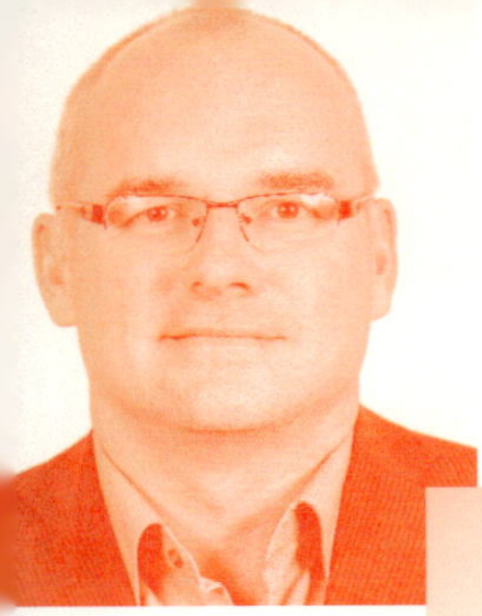
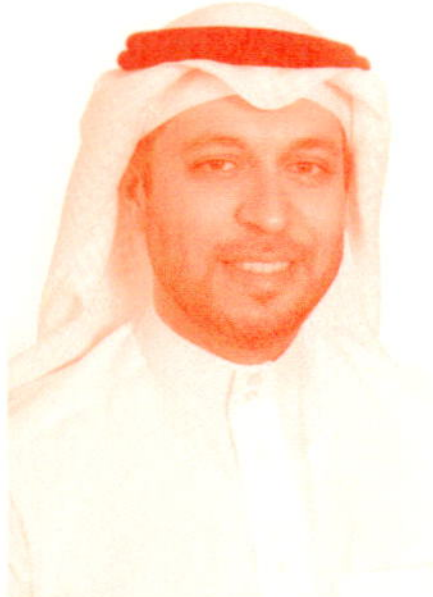
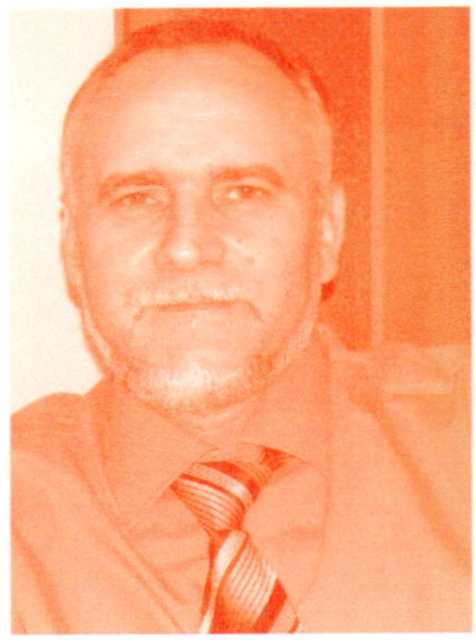
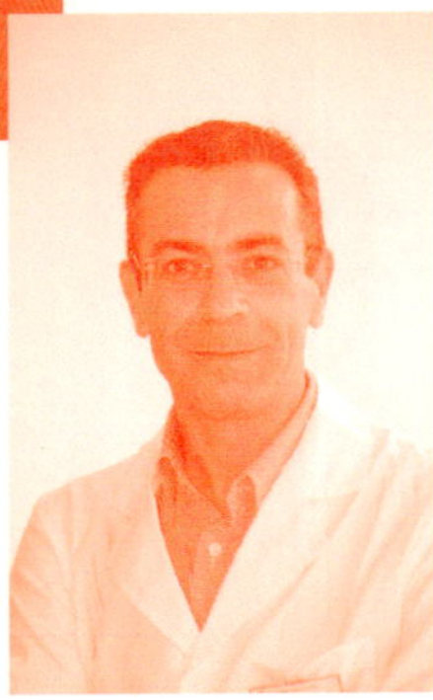
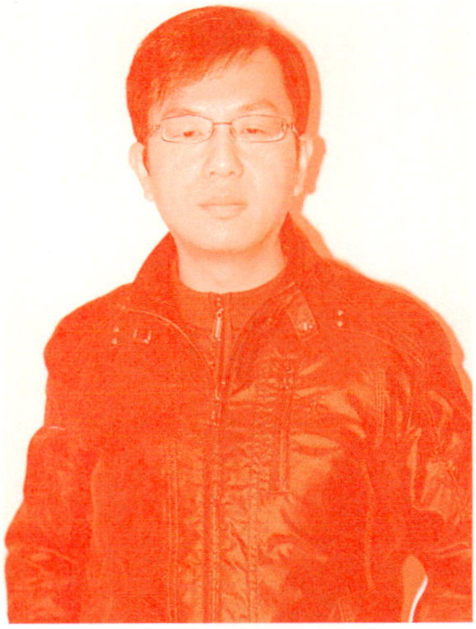
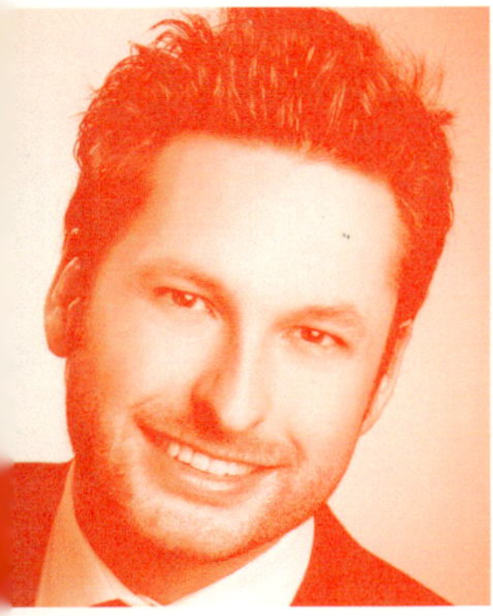
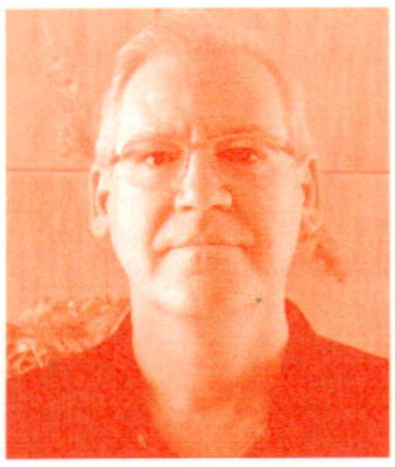

IntechOpen

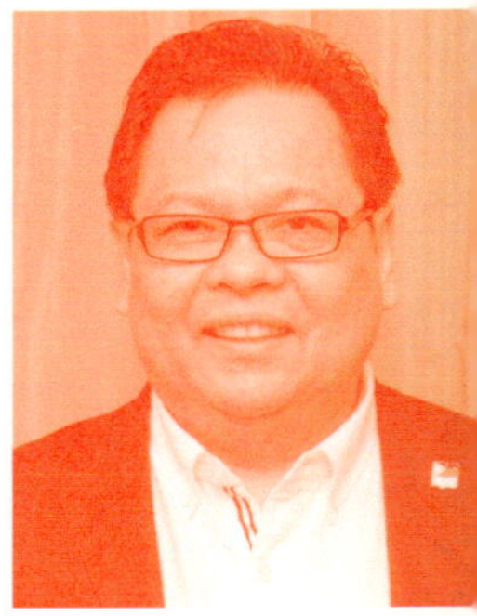
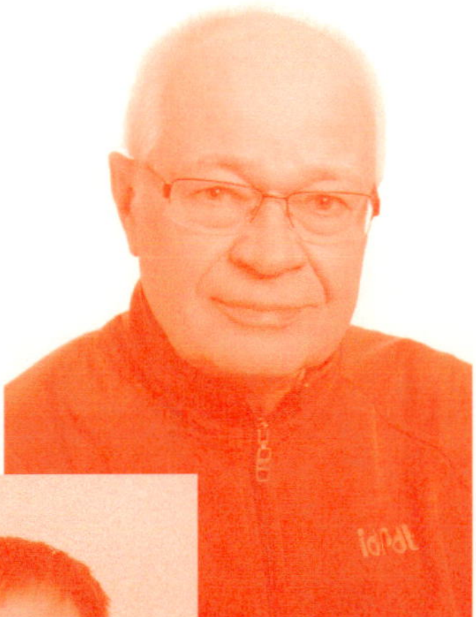
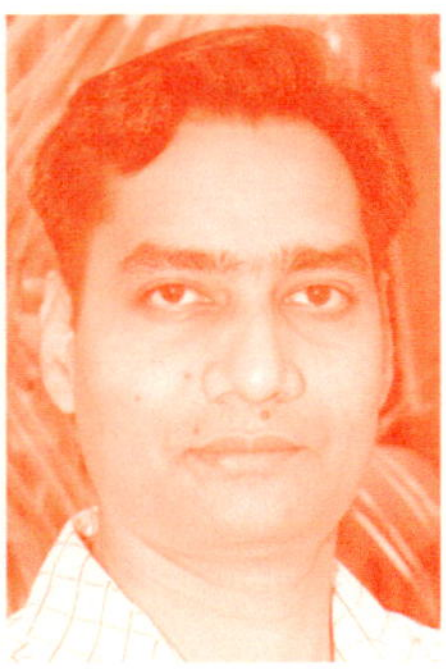
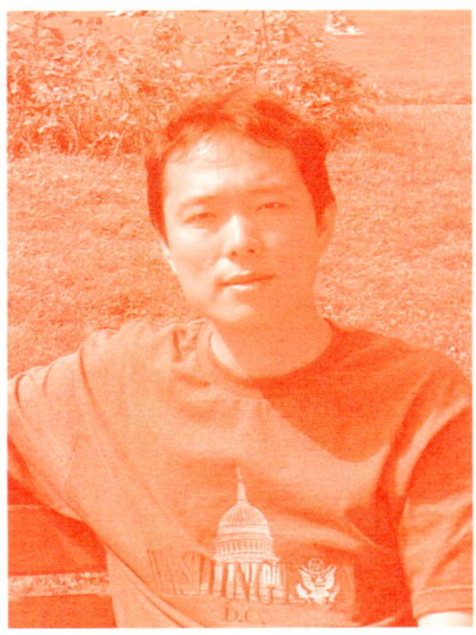
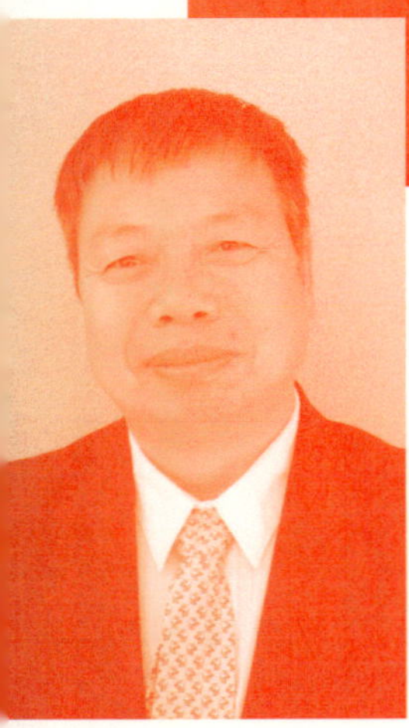
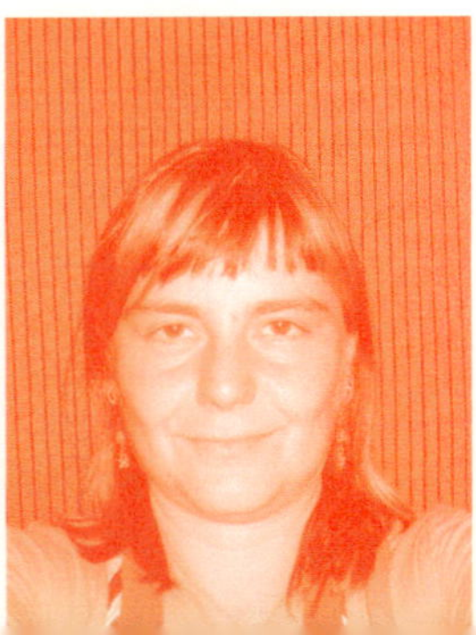

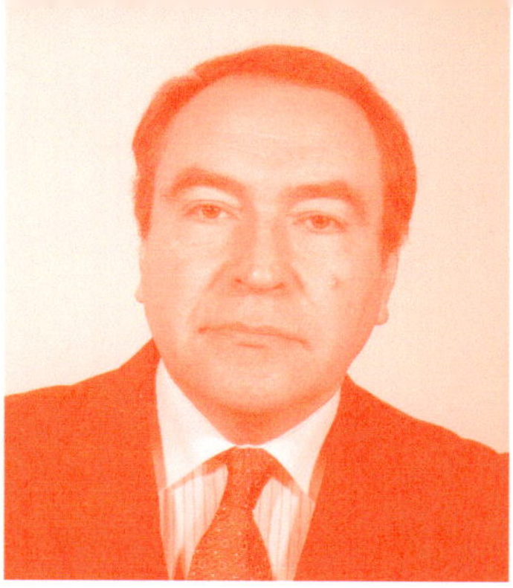
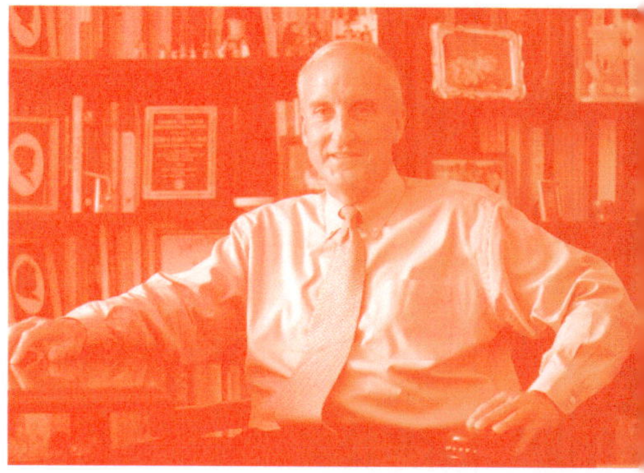
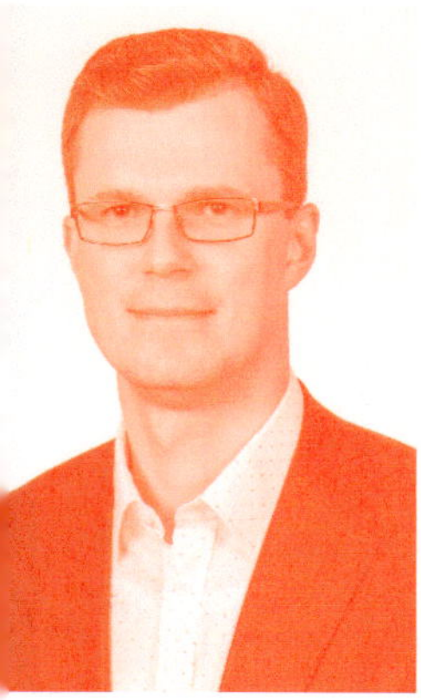
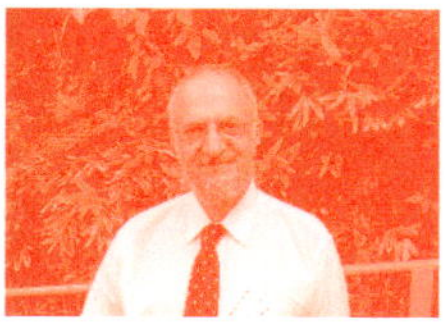
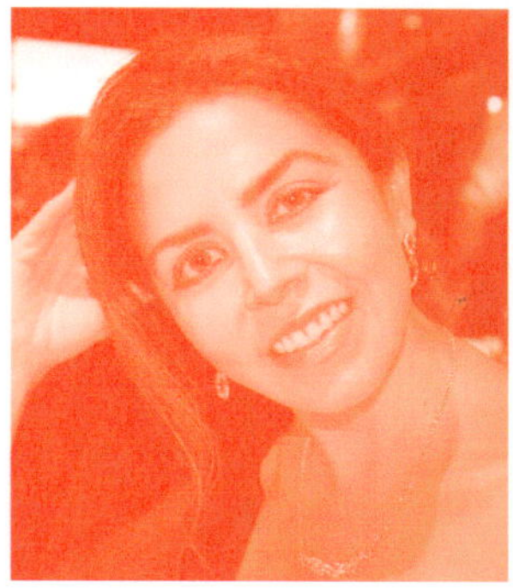

Supporting open minds since 2005

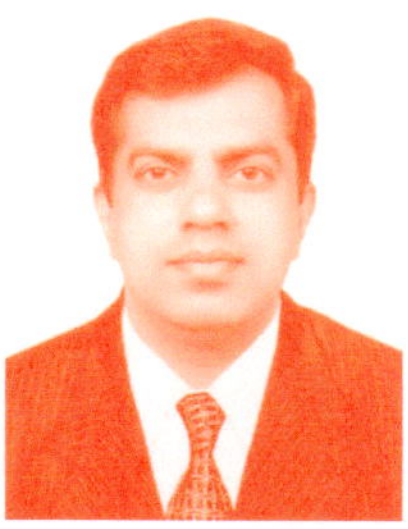
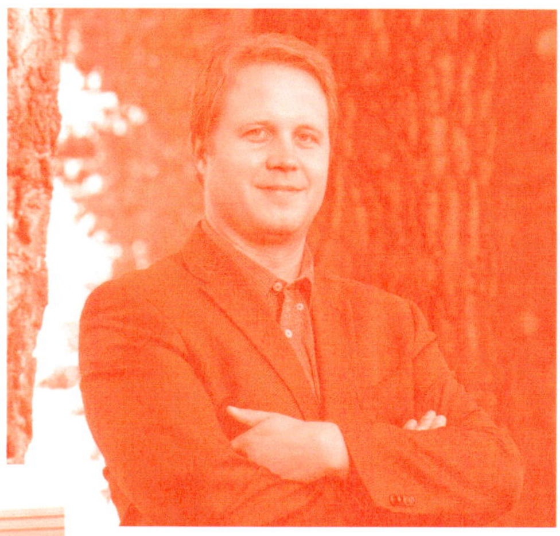
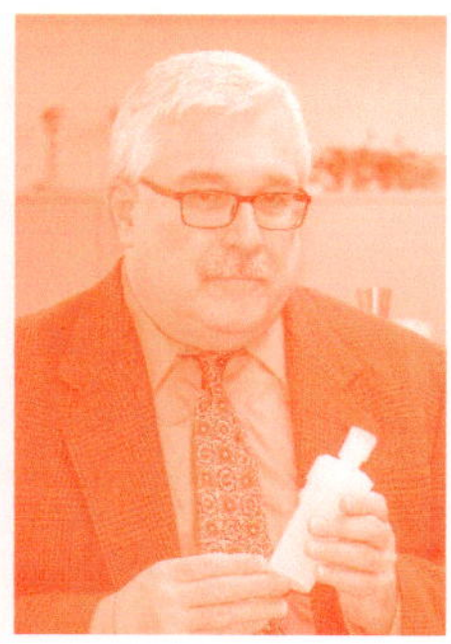
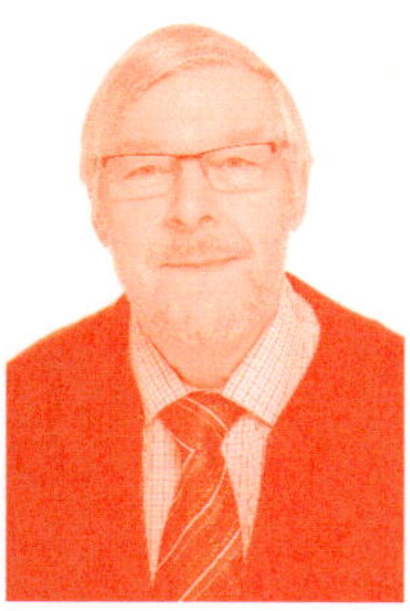
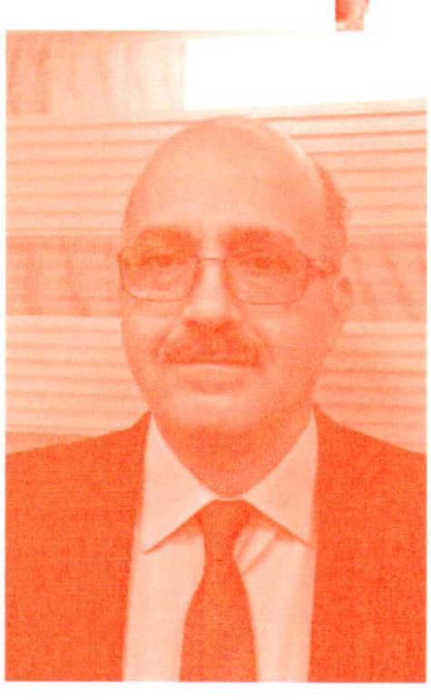
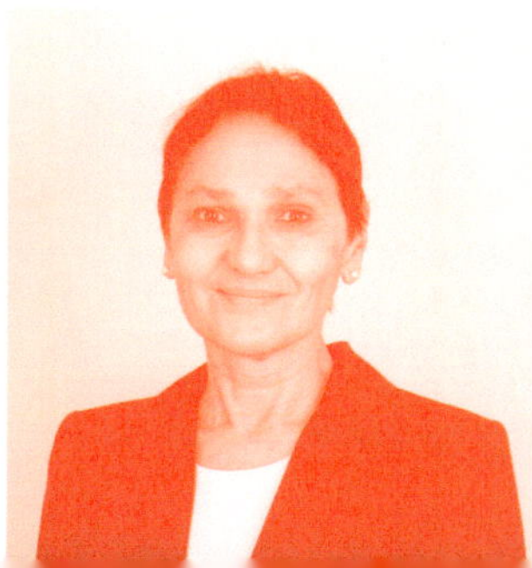
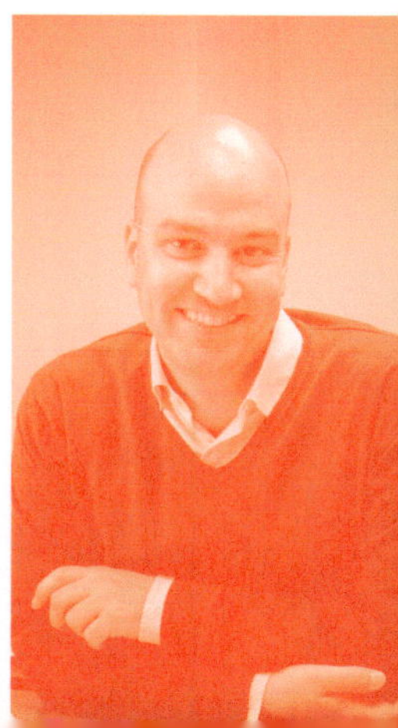

Overview on Echinococcosis
http://dx.doi.org/10.5772/intechopen.77811
Edited by Fethi Derbel and Meriem Braiki

Part of IntechOpen Book Series: Infectious Diseases, Volume 6
Book Series Editor: Shailendra K. Saxena

Contributors
Pedro Pablo Pinto Guerrero, Sergio Gaete, Tuba Apaydın, Irina Magdalena Dumitru, Fethi Derbel, Meriem Braiki, Azzaza Mohamed, Rebecca Weka, Pam Luka, Ndudim Ogo, Paul Weka, Triwibowo Ambar Garjito, Mohammad Sudomo, Mujiyanto Mujiyanto, Khadeeja Abees Al-Khalidi, Mehmet Mihmanli, Mert Tanal, Emre Bozkurt, Onur Guven

First published in London, United Kingdom, 2020 by IntechOpen
IntechOpen is the global imprint of INTECHOPEN LIMITED, registered in England and Wales, registration number: 11086078, 7th floor, 10 Lower Thames Street, London, EC3R 6AF, United Kingdom
Printed in Croatia

British Library Cataloguing-in-Publication Data
A catalogue record for this book is available from the British Library

Additional hard and PDF copies can be obtained from orders@intechopen.com

Overview on Echinococcosis
Edited by Fethi Derbel and Meriem Braiki
p. cm.
Print ISBN 978-1-83880-478-7
Online ISBN 978-1-83880-479-4
eBook (PDF) ISBN 978-1-83880-482-4
ISSN 2631-6188

For EU product safety concerns:
IN TECH d.o.o., Prolaz Marije Krucifikse Kozulić 3, 51000 Rijeka, Croatia, info@intechopen.com or visit our website at intechopen.com.

IntechOpen Book Series

Infectious Diseases

Volume 6

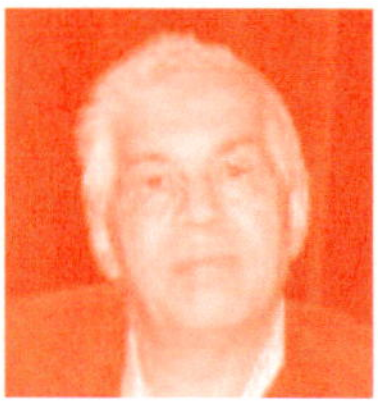

Professor Fethi Derbel was born in 1960 in Tunisia. He received his medical degree from the Faculty of Medicine in Sousse, Tunisia. He completed his surgical residency in General Surgery at the University Hospital Farhat Hached (Sousse) and was a member of the Unit of Liver Transplantation at the University of Rennes, France. He is currently working at the Les Oliviers private clinic. His hospital activities are mostly concerned with laparoscopic, colorectal, pancreatic, hepato-biliary and gastric surgery. He has worked as a professor of Medicine in Djibouti, was a past member of the medical committee in the University Hospital Sahloul, Sousse and a member of the National College of Surgeons in Tunisia. He has published many articles in journals and collaborates intensively with IntechOpen as an editor.

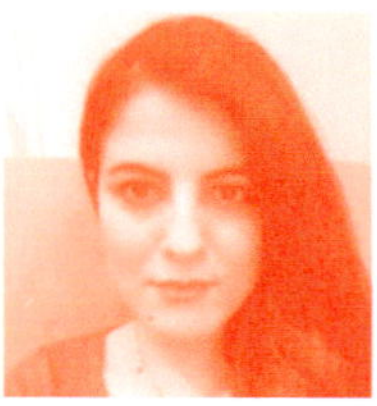

Dr Meriem Braiki is a specialist in pediatric surgery from Tunisia. She was born in 1985. She received her medical degree from the University of Medicine at Sousse, Tunisia. She achieved her surgical residency training periods in the Pediatric Surgery departments at university hospitals in Monastir, Tunis and France. She is currently working in the Pediatric Surgery Department, Sidi Bouzid Hospital, Tunisia. Her hospital activities are mostly concerned with laparoscopic, parietal, urological and digestive surgery. She has published several articles in different journals.

Editors of Volume 6:
Professor Fethi Derbel
Les Oliviers Private Clinic, Tunisia

Meriem Braiki
Sidi Bouzid Regional Hospital, Tunisia

Book Series Editor:
Shailendra K. Saxena
King George's Medical University

Scope of the Series

The series will give a most comprehensive overview of recent trends in various infectious diseases (as per the most recent Baltimore classification), as well as general concepts of infections, immunopathology, diagnosis, treatment, epidemiology and etiology to current clinical recommendations in management of infectious diseases, highlighting the ongoing issues, recent advances, with future directions in diagnostic approaches and therapeutic strategies. This book series will focus on various aspects and properties of infectious diseases whose deep understanding is very important for safeguarding human race from more loss of resources and economies due to pathogens.

Contents

Preface

We are very pleased to present this book dealing with echinococcosis.

The chapters in this book are written by surgeons, radiologists and parasitologists from different hospitals in several countries as Tunisia, Turkey, Indonesia, Nigeria, Romania, Chile and Iraq.

The book is subdivided into five sections and eight chapters:

1. Introductory chapter, overview on Echinococcosis.

2. Epidemiology

3. Parasitology

4. Imaging

5. Treatment

I would like to congratulate all the authors of this book and their teams for the quality of the chapters. I highly recommend this book to all clinicians, radiologists, internists and surgeons involved in the management of patients with echinococcosis.

As editor of this book, I would like to acknowledge the effort made by all the contributing authors and the entire editorial team in the publishing of this book, especially Ms Mia Vulovic for her precious collaboration.

Special thanks to Dr Meriem Braiki, pediatric surgeon, for her valuable collaboration as co-editor and her great help in revising the manuscripts.

Finally, I thank the authors of these excellent articles. They were willing to share their knowledge with a wider audience. I enjoyed working with them, getting to know them and learning from them. I apologize to those friends whose names I may have overlooked.

I would like to dedicate this book to all my colleagues, surgeons, radiologists, internists and parasitologists. I also dedicate it especially to Dr Ridha Ben Haj Hmida, Rached Letaief, Ali Ben Ali, Jaafar Mazhoud, Sabri Youssef, Mohamed Ben Mabrouk, Younes Dahmene, Mohamed Azzaza and Mehdi Ben Haj Hmida. These surgeons have vast experience in the management of echinococcosis.

Fethi Derbel
Professor,
Les Oliviers Private Clinic,
Tunisia

Meriem Braiki
Sidi Bouzid Regional Hospital,
Tunisia

Section 1

Introduction

Chapter 1

Introductory Chapter: Overview on Echinococcosis

Meriem Braiki, Azzaza Mohamed and Fethi Derbel

1. Introduction

Echinococcosis is considered the most common parasitic disease and the most widespread zoonotic infection caused by several cestode species belonging to the genus *Echinococcus* [1].

This parasite has 12 different genus types, though four major species are known to cause human parasitic disease: *Echinococcus granulosus* (*E. granulosus*), *Echinococcus multilocularis*, *Echinococcus vogeli*, and *Echinococcus oligarthrus* [2].

E. granulosus is the causative organism of cystic echinococcosis, a small-sized tapeworm measuring approximately 2–7 mm in length with at least 10 different genome patterns and distinct genetic markers [1].

2. Parasitology

The parasitic life cycle involves two mammalian hosts. The intermediate hosts include members of the ungulates such as sheep, goats, and pigs. The definitive host of this parasite is the dog and other members of canids.

The adult parasite inhabits the small intestine of a definitive host and eggs, containing infective oncospheres, are produced. Subsequently, free eggs as well as cestode segments are excreted through the stool of the host into the environment [1].

Following an oral uptake of eggs by an intermediate host, a larval stage (metacestode) develops in several internal organs, mainly the liver and lungs, after a larval migration through the blood and lymph vessels. Typically, numerous protoscoleces are produced by the mature metacestode, each with the potential to develop into an adult cestode after oral ingestion by a suitable definitive host [3].

Humans are accidental or aberrant hosts that are not essential to the natural *Echinococcus* life-cycle. The eggs, after being ingested, develop as a cyst (hydatid cyst) inside the accidental host organs. Larval infection leading to the hydatid disease is characterized by metacestode long-term growth in the intermediate host. The parasitic cystic structure is typically filled with a clear hydatid fluid [4]. The inner germinating membrane of the cyst provides germination and the outer cystic layer features a laminated part. A granulomatous inflammatory reaction leads to a fibrous tissue constitution walling the cyst [5].

Developing cysts are responsible for the morbidity and the mortality related to the disease [3].

Cystic echinococcosis (CE) occurs worldwide. *E. granulosus* is known to occur on all continents but high parasite prevalences are found in endemic areas such as central Asia, the Mediterranean Basin, the Russian Federation, Africa (northern and eastern regions), Australia, and South America [1, 3].

IntechOpen

Although Echinococcosis is regarded as an eradicable disease, it leads to serious economic losses for public health systems and agricultural sectors in endemic areas [6]. Therefore, numerous control programs reveal that preventive measures for the interruption of parasitic life cycle may relatively reduce the prevalence and the incidence of the hydatid disease [3, 7].

3. Diagnosis

3.1 Clinic

CE clinical presentation reflects the presence of one or more unilocular fluid-filled cysts. Liver and lungs are most commonly affected: about 70% of cysts involve the liver and the lungs are involved in 20% followed by other organs such as spleen, kidney, brain, breasts, and bone.

The disease course is typically slow and most patients have an asymptomatic disease course for several years. Otherwise, the cystic slow growth rate is estimated at 1–5 mm per year and patients develop symptoms as the cyst gradually grows [5, 8–10].

In the early stage of echinococcosis, clinical manifestations are mild. At later stages, damaged tissues and organs can become dysfunctional with the occurrence of symptoms related to cystic complications.

Symptoms are nonspecific and the diagnosis is often incidental, based on immunological tests and imaging such as standard radiology, ultrasonography (US), computed axial tomography (CT), and magnetic resonance imaging (MRI).

3.2 Serology

Serologic diagnostic methods play an important complementary role. They are used in order to support the radiological diagnosis and for follow-up of patients after surgical or pharmacological management.

There are multiple immunological responses to the disease. Mild immune response is noted with rugged and intact cysts, whereas complicated cysts (leaking or ruptured cysts) tend to show a strong immune response [4].

Serodiagnosis consists of the detection of specific serum antibodies by multiple immunodiagnostic tests. An optimum test should be specific with high sensitivity. There are considerable differences between the various serological tests, concerning the specificity as well as the test sensitivity.

In routine laboratory applications, the indirect hemagglutination (IHA) is often nonspecific, while the enzyme-linked immunosorbent assay (ELISA) using crude hydatid cyst fluid has a high sensitivity (up to 95%) with low specificity. Concomitant use of both tests (IHA and ELISA) is associated with diagnostic sensitivity over than 85–96% [1, 11].

False-positive serological findings are revealed in 20% of patients with CE, which is mainly related to cross-reactions with other parasitic diseases. Furthermore, seronegativity rate is relatively higher in cases with nonactive disease stages, in patients treated for autoimmune or malignant pathologies and during pregnancy [12]. Cysts in the bone, brain and calcified cysts often show no or low immunological response [5].

Immunoblot analysis is generally used when IHA and ELISA findings are not definitive. The immunological diagnosis is established by the detection of specific serum antibodies. Immunological methods often use the most specific antigens: *E. granulosus*, antigen B, and antigen 5 (Ag5) [1, 13].

3.3 Imaging

US is considered as the first choice imaging modality in the diagnosis and follow-up. It is a convenient and efficient imaging tool that demonstrates the cystic number, location, and size. Furthermore, US can guide the interventional radiology, which is often available, safe, and cost-efficient method with no radiation. Therefore, it can be used in endemic areas with large populations to make a prompt diagnosis. It mainly explores abdominal location.

Typically, the liver involvement is shown as a mixed echogenic, heterogeneous pattern with irregular contours with multiple distributed calcific foci, whereas, the radiologist must be aware of differential diagnosis in less typical appearance. The criteria for ultrasonographic cystic classification of liver was first made by Gharbi in 1981, and then, improved by the World Health Organization (WHO) in 2001 [5]. Cysts in other sites like the brain and the lung are not well demonstrated with US and it require the use of other screening techniques. Conventional radiography can be required as the initial imaging modality to diagnose thoracic and bone involvement. The X-ray findings are nonspecific and are visualized as multiple small opacities [14].

CT and MRI are mainly used in some cases, where US does not provide definitive findings. These imaging tools are necessary for illustrating the lesions morphologic features in intra-abdominal organs, which are involved through a direct invasion from the primary lesion or disseminated disease.

They are also indicated in patients with sub-diaphragmatic location, extra-abdominal sites (in bone and soft tissues involvement), complicated cysts such as cysto-biliary fistulae and abscess, cases with extra-abdominal dissemination. Moreover, CT and MRI can be useful for the preoperative evaluation and for patient's follow-up examination.

The radiologist should be familiar with multimodality imaging findings of this particular disease. Thus, according to the organ involvement, the lesion can be confused with other differential diagnosis including neoplasms, metastatic neoplasms, or abscess [14].

4. Treatment

There are several treatment approaches for echinococcosis, including monitoring (watch and wait strategy), chemotherapy, interventional radiology, and surgery. Indications for one or more management options are complex and depend on the cyst features, medical and surgical equipment availability and the patient's cooperation. Therefore, it is preferable to refer patients to reference treatment centers for echinococcosis in order to get the suitable management [15].

4.1 Medical treatment

The choice of the therapeutic modality is related to cyst stage, size, site, and comorbidities.

Medical treatment using parasitostatic drugs such as benzimidazoles (mebendazole and albendazole) is mainly recommended for inoperable patients and patients with disseminated disease. Drug therapy should be administered continuously for at least 3 months. However, prolonged treatment has a high cost with multiple teratogenic side effects [16]. Moreover, chemotherapy can be used as a complementary therapy to surgery or to prevent metastasis and secondary cystic sites. However, it is not recommended in the treatment of inactive or calcified cysts [17].

The watch and wait strategy is a therapeutic option for uncomplicated cysts with multiple involvements. It requires a regular long-term monitoring of liver function tests and leukocyte counts [17].

4.2 Percutaneous treatment

The percutaneous treatment modality is defined as an option for the management of cysts in the liver and other abdominal locations. This procedure is divided into two techniques: (1) PAIR technique is the best known, consisting of the destruction of the germinal membrane following the use of a scolicidal agent and (2) modified catheterization techniques aiming at the entire endocyst evacuation. This approach is a mini invasive procedure comparing to the surgery, but cysts containing daughter vesicles are not the best indication for percutaneous treatment because of the high risk of spread into the peritoneal cavity and into the biliary tract [5].

4.3 Surgical treatment

Surgery should be carefully evaluated. The decision-making is based on the characteristics of the hydatid cyst as the cyst type, number, size, location, and the presence or not of associated complications. It is well recommended for large cysts containing multiple daughter vesicles, symptomatic and complicated cysts, cysts with superficial location that may be ruptured spontaneously or following a benign trauma, infected cysts and cysts with close contact with vessels or adjacent vital organs. Furthermore, it can be an option for patients not suitable for percutaneous treatment.

The surgical approach is aiming to parasite inactivation, evacuation of the endocyst with the prevention of contamination, germinal layer removal, and residual cavity management [18].

Regarding the abdominal sites (typically the hepatic involvement), there are two surgical approaches consisting of a conservative surgery and radical procedure using open or laparoscopic surgery [19].

Conservative procedures consist of the parasitic cyst contents removal such as daughter vesicles and germinative membrane, whereas the pericyst is retained. The residual cavity is carefully explored to research any evidence of cystic biliary tract communication and then managed according to different techniques: capitonnage, omentoplasty, or external drainage.

Surgeons should cover the operating field with a scolicidal agent in order to avoid the parasites spillage and the peritoneal cavity contamination.

Conservative surgery is simple, safe with relatively reduced operative time, but has high morbidity and recurrence rates [19].

Radical surgery is the first therapeutic choice suitable for total excision of the entire parasitic lesion. Whenever possible, complete resection is required because radical surgical procedures are superior to conservative surgical methods and may cure definitively the patient [18].

The radical surgery target is the removal of the whole cyst with the parasitic contents and pericystic tissue.

Radical procedures includes: partial cystectomy, total cystic removal through an open or closed pericystectomy, and hepatic resection.

During the pericystectomy, a proper cleavage plane between the inner layer and the outer cystic layer may limit the liver parenchyma damage.

Hepatic resection is more difficult, takes longer operative time with higher risk of blood loss but lower cystic recurrence rates.

Comparing to conservative treatment, radical surgery is preferable due to lower morbidity, mortality, and reoccurrence rates [19].

Laparoscopic management of hydatid cysts with abdominal (hepatic or extra-hepatic sites) has its place among management approaches. It is a mini invasive surgery that can be safely achieved in particular cases after patients' selection.

Laparoscopy has several advantages including: better visualization of the peritoneal cavity and internal organs, prompt postoperative discharge, limited postoperative morbidity, and good esthetic outcomes [18].

There is lower frequency of hydatid disease in extra-hepatic sites. The management and the proper therapeutic approach depend essentially on cystic site and the organ involved. Generally, when the removal of the cysts is complete, the prognosis is good with low rate of recurrence [20].

5. Follow-up

A long-term follow-up for patients managed for hydatid disease should be planned because recurrences may occur in some cases. The patient monitoring is mainly based on imaging techniques (US, CT, and MRI) at short intervals. Serological tools and specific serum antibodies dosage support imaging techniques and can reflect metastode viability. Moreover, the monitoring of parasitostatic plasma level is necessary to adjust the therapeutic range and to prevent long-term treatment side effects [20].

Currently, planning for the echinococcosis control relies on the interruption of parasitic life cycle. The disease can be prevented by hygiene improvement in the slaughtering of livestock, public education campaigns, periodic deworming of dogs, and adequate destruction of infected offal. Vaccination of dogs with recombinant proteins provides encouraging prospects for prevention and control [21].

Author details

Meriem Braiki[1], Azzaza Mohamed[2] and Fethi Derbel[3]*

1 Department of Surgery, Sidi Bouzid Hospital, Tunisia

2 Department of Surgery, Sahloul University Hospital, Sousse, Tunisia

3 Department of Surgery, Clinic "Les Olivier", Sousse, Tunisia

*Address all correspondence to: fethi.derbel@gmail.com

References

[1] Eckert J, Deplazes P. Biological, epidemiological, and clinical aspects of echinococcosis, a zoonosis of increasing concern. Clinical Microbiology Reviews. 2004;**17**:107-135

[2] Nascimento G, Silva C, Marques R, Silva C, Oliveira JF, Santos J, et al. Periprosthetic pathologic fracture following tibial echinoccocosis: A case report. International Journal of Surgery Case Reports. 2018;**51**:231-236

[3] Lopez-Bernus A, Belhassen-García M, Carpio-Perez A, Perez del Villar L, Romero-Alegria A, Velasco-Tirado V, et al. Is cystic echinoccocosis re-emerging in western Spain? Epidemiology and Infection. 2015;**143**:3351-3357

[4] Zhang W, McManus DP. Recent advances in the immunology and diagnosis of echinococcosis. FEMS Immunology and Medical Microbiology. 2006;**47**:24-41

[5] Gharbi HA, Hassine W, Brauner MW, Dupuch K. Ultrasound examination of the hydatic liver. Radiology. 1981;**139**(2):459-463

[6] Budke CM, Deplazes P, Torgerson PR. Global socioeconomic impact of cystic echinococcosis. Emerging Infectious Diseases. 2006;**12**:296-303

[7] Jiménez S et al. Progress in control of cystic echinococcosis in La Rioja, Spain: Decline in infection prevalences in human and animal hosts and economic costs and benefits. Acta Tropica. 2002;**83**:213-221

[8] Nunnari G, Pinzone MR, Gruttadauria S, Celesia BM, Madeddu G, Malaguarnera G, et al. Hepatic echinococcosis: Clinical and therapeutic aspects. World Journal of Gastroenterology. 2012;**18**:1448-1458

[9] Rinaldi F, Brunetti E, Neumayr A, Maestri M, Goblirsch S, Tamarozzi F. Cystic echinococcosis of the liver: A primer for hepatologists. World Journal of Hepatology. 2014;**6**:293-305

[10] Moro P, Schantz PM. Echinococcosis: A review. International Journal of Infectious Diseases. 2009;**13**:125-133

[11] Deplazes P, Eckert J. Veterinary aspects of alveolar echinococcosis—A zoonosis of public health significance. Veterinary Parasitology. 2001;**98**:65-87

[12] Wuestenberg J, Gruener B, Oeztuerk S, Mason RA, Haenle MM, Graeter T, et al. Diagnostics in cystic echinococcosis: Serology versus ultrasonography. The Turkish Journal of Gastroenterology. 2014;**25**:398-404

[13] Ito A, Sako Y, Yamasaki H, Mamuti W, Nakaya K, Nakao M, et al. Development of Em18-immoblot and Em18-ELISA for specific diagnosis of alveolar echinococcosis. Acta Tropica. 2003;**85**:173-182

[14] Bulakçı M, Kartal MG, Yılmaz S, Yılmaz E, Yılmaz R, Şahin D, et al. Multimodality imaging in diagnosis and management of alveolar echinococcosis: An update. Diagnostic and Interventional Radiology. 2016;**22**:247-256

[15] Ilica AT, Kocaoglu M, Zeybek N, Guven S, Adaletli I, Basgul A, et al. Extrahepatic abdominal hydatid disease caused by *Echinococcus granulosus*: Imaging findings. American Journal of Roentgenology. 2007;**189**:337-343

[16] Velasco-Tirado V, Alonso-Sardón M, Lopez-Bernus A, Romero-Alegría Á, Burguillo FJ, Muro A, et al. Medical treatment of cystic echinococcosis: Systematic review and meta-analysis. BMC Infectious Diseases. 2018;**18**:306

[17] Nazligul Y, Kucukazman M, Akbulut S. Role of chemotherapeutic agents in the management of cystic echinococcosis. International Surgery. 2015;**100**:112-114

[18] Thota A, Reddy AD, Venkata Narasimha Rao V. Surgical treatment of abdominal echinococcosis. International Surgery Journal. 2018;**5**(12)

[19] Vidoura A, Parisidou M, Chatedaki C, Zacharoulis D. Surgical Management of Hydatid Disease. Rijeka, Croatia: IntechOpen;

[20] Brunettia E, Kern P, Vuitton DA. Expert consensus for the diagnosis and treatment of cystic and alveolar echinococcosis in humans. Acta Tropica. 2010;**114**:1-16

[21] Otero-Abad B, Torgerson PR. A systematic review of the epidemiology of echinococcosis in domestic and wild animals. PLoS Neglected Tropical Diseases. 2013;7(6):2249

Section 2

Epidemiology

Chapter 2

Echinococcosis: Past and Present Situation in Southeast Asia

Triwibowo Ambar Garjito, Mujiyanto Mujiyanto and Mohammad Sudomo

Abstract

In Asia, Southeast Asia is reported as a non-endemic area of the parasite. However, several indigenous echinococcoses in human and animals were reported in several countries, such as Malaysia, Thailand, the Philippines, Indonesia, Vietnam, Cambodia, and Lao People's Democratic Republic (PDR). Most human infections are caused by *Echinococcus granulosus* and only two cases with *E. ortleppi*. There was no evidence case with *E. multilocularis* in Southeast Asia. *Echinococcus granulosus* infection is prevalent in areas that association with dogs and livestocks that close contact with dogs. The incidence is very low. A total of 49 cases of echinococcosis was identified in Southeast Asia from 1885 to 2015. Of which, at least 31 cases were indigenous, 14 cases were imported, and 4 cases were unknown. Thailand is the most prevalent country with echinococcosis in human, followed by very low incidence in Indonesia, Malaysia, Vietnam, the Philippines, Cambodia and Lao PDR. However, it is very difficult to estimate the real number of human echinococcosis case in Southeast Asia due to the long asymptomatic period that is usually >5 years. The disease may be more prevalent in Southeast Asia; however, they were underdiagnosed and not reported.

Keywords: echinococcosis, Southeast Asia, *Echinococcus granulosus*, *Echinococcus ortleppi*, incidence

1. Introduction

Echinococcosis (hydatidosis) is one of the neglected zoonosis caused by adult or larval stage of the cestodes belonging to the genus *Echinococcus* of the family Taeniidae [1–3]. At least nine species of *Echinococcus* have been recognized, including *Echinococcus granulosus* sensu stricto (GI [sheep strain], G2 [Tasmanian sheep strain], G3 [buffalo strain]), *E. equinus* (G4), *E. ortleppi* (G5), *E. canadensis* (G6–G10), *E. vogeli*, *E. oligarthrus*, *E. multilocularis*, *E. shiquicus* and *E. felidis*. Three among them, *E. granulosus*, *E. multilocularis*, and *E. ortleppi*, have a medical importance and cause alveolar echinococcosis (AE) and cystic echinococcosis (CE) [4–6]. Human alveolar echinococcosis has limited distribution in the northern hemisphere, while cystic echinococcosis is more widely distributed and cosmopolitan, particularly in countries of the temperate zones.

Southeast Asia is reported as non-endemic area of the parasite. However, several indigenous echinococcoses in human and animals were reported in several countries, such as Malaysia, Thailand, the Philippines, Indonesia, Vietnam, Cambodia, and Lao People's Democratic Republic (PDR). Although the surveillance of echinococcosis was not routinely conducted in several countries and the cases were scarcely reported in Southeast Asia. In the recent years, by clinical, radiological, microscopic, and serological aspects, the disease was found in many areas in this region. This situation makes us alert on the possibility of echinococcosis as one of the potential health problems in the Southeast Asia.

2. Indonesia

Human echinococcosis in Indonesia was first reported in nonindigenous people, in a European with liver hydatidosis in 1885 [7]. Subsequent cases were also confirmed in four European and an Indian in the 1920s [8]. In the late 1930s, a 45-year-old European female was also suspected with *Echinococcus* infection after stayed for almost 17 years which much contact with dogs in Indonesia [9].

The first indigenous case was diagnosed in a female aged 23 years from the northern part of South Sulawesi in 1988. She was admitted to the hospital with pain in the right under quadrant of the abdomens and in the right part of the hypochondrium, below the right rib. Hepatomegaly or tumor in the right upper quadrant of the abdomen was not found by physical examination. However, a hypoechoic, oval image, with a clear acoustic image on the right, was identified by using ultrasonography. Serological test was not performed, and the diagnosis was confirmed by radiological image examination. The patient has a history of keeping a dog [10].

Another echinococcosis case was reported in a 90-year-old female from Java in 1988. She was hospitalized in Ujung Pandang (Makassar), South Sulawesi with complaint of severe weakness, fainting, and no appetite. A tumor with no malignant cells was identified in the lower right part of the abdomen. Cysts with hypoechoic image on the walls were detected in the pelvis, right upper liver, and upper left abdomen. Fluid aspiration and serological test were not carried out during patient treatment at the hospital. The hydatidosis was confirmed in the right diaphragm arc/liver, omentum, and adnexa by radio-image. She had not kept dog at home [11].

In 1997, subsequent indigenous case, a 26-year-old female from Palu, Central Sulawesi, was administered in the Cipto Mangunkusumo Hospital in Jakarta with chronic and progressive headache, space-occupying lesion, blurred vision since the last 6 months, and vomiting. Bilateral edema of the papilla of the eyes was found without other neurological deficits. Cysts were found in many parts of organs. A hypodense, cystic lesion in the left parietal region of the brain divided by several septa with calcifications was discovered by radio-image with tomography (CT) scan. Historically, he lived in an area that kept many dogs, including her house.

In animals, echinococcosis is reported from goat, sheep, pig, water buffalo, and monkey from Sumatra, Madura, Bali, and Sulawesi. A case with liver, lung, and spleen hydatidosis was first identified in a cattle in Buitenzorg (Bogor, West Java) during meat inspection on 1906. Hydatid cysts were subsequently found from the lungs and liver of cattle in North Sumatra in 1907 [12]. At that time, the hydatid cysts were only detected from imported Australian cattles (nonindigenous echinococcosis was also reported among 46 cattles and 3 pigs in Medan, North Sumatra, in 1916) [13]. In 1929, hydatid cysts in indigenous cattle were found for the first time from Bali. This finding was considered that dogs from Bali were probably reservoirs for the adult worm *Echinococcus granulosus*. However, the lack of study has caused this to never to be proven [14]. Further cases of echinococcosis in animals were reported back in 1940. A single cyst of *Echinococcus* was found in the lung of the goat (*Capra hircus*) and the lung of the buffalo (*Buffelus sondaicus*) in the

Netherlands Indies [15]. In 1947, a total of 45 cysts of *Echinococcus unilocularis* (*E. granulosus*) were found in the lungs, kidney, stomach wall, and liver on an old monkey *Cynopithecus niger* (later on as *Macaca tonkeana*) from Sulawesi (Celebes) that suddenly died. The first evidence of *E. granulosus* infection in domestic dogs in Indonesia was reported from the Lindu Valley, Central Sulawesi, in 1972. The dog died suddenly after 18 months with numerous necropsies due to *E. granulosus*. Subsequent dog with echinococcosis was reported on the shore of Lake Lindu at Tomado village in 1973. The positive eggs of *E. granulosus* were confirmed by direct smear and formaldehyde-ether from the dog stools. The adult worms of *E. granulosus* were also identified during the study. The worms were collected from a dead dog on the shore of Lake Lindu at Tomado [16]. Since then, hundreds of dogs have been examined to identify the infection rate of *E. granulosus* in this area. However, hydatid cysts and adult *E. granulosus* have not been discovered until now [13].

3. Thailand

In Thailand, at least 18 reports of echinococcosis were confirmed in indigenous Thai population, 5 cases were recorded from imported echinococcosis, and other 4 cases were noted with unknown origin during 1936–2007 [17–19]. Almost all cases were recorded as cystic echinococcosis, and only two cases were identified as alveolar echinococcosis [20–25]. Indigenous cases are distributed from the northern, central, and southern regions of Thailand [17–19].

The disease infection was reported for the first time in this country in 1936 from a 52-year-old male with peritoneum infection in Chiang Mai. The patient finally died due to severe infection without surgical removal and antiparasitic drug [25]. Subsequently, human case of echinococcosis was found in a 16-year-old male with *E. granulosus* cysts infection in lung in 1952. He is an Indian citizen who previously lived in India. He was diagnosed with echinococcosis while in Bangkok [20]. Another patient, a Thai female, aged 56 years, with lung infection was confirmed to be echinococcosis in 1980 [26]. Infection of *E. granulosus* cysts in the lung is a common manifestation in Thailand. Five other cases of lung echinococcosis, two females and three males with an age range of 32–71 years old, were also confirmed in between 1980 and 1995 [17, 18, 20–22, 27, 28]. Surgical removals were performed in all patients, and two of them received antiparasitic drug treatment with albendazole. Two cases with renal echinococcosis were subsequently reported in a 39-year-old woman in 1993 and 43-year-old man in 1997. The first patient has recovered after marsupialization; however the second patient died several years after infection and treatment in 2000 [18, 29].

The most frequent echinococcosis case in this country is liver infection. At least 12 cases were reported in the period 1960–2007 [18, 19, 23, 27, 30, 31]. Two cases, 50-year-old male and 50-year-old female, were reported as Thai citizens who had a history of visiting the Middle East in 1994 and 1996, respectively [17, 18], while the other two were identified from non-Thai citizens who previously lived in Middle East countries. Middle East countries are known as an endemic area of echinococcosis.

Liver echinococcosis was also reported in a Thai citizen who had a history of traveling to Switzerland in 2004. One subsequent case was recognized as a Nepali citizen who was visiting Thailand in 1995, while three cases were recorded as unknown origin in 1994 and 2004 [30]. In 2007, two cases were reported with echinococcal cystic mass in the liver that was diagnosed through serological testing using an indirect enzyme-linked immunosorbent assay (ELISA) [19]. Physical examination revealed that hepatomegaly or tumor in the right upper quadrant of the abdomen was detected in almost all of liver echinococcosis cases [19, 23, 27].

The hydatid cysts were also found in the jaw and foot. One case with foot echinococcosis was reported in a Thai 45-year-old female from Nakhon Pathom province in 1989, while jaw echinococcosis was identified in a male, aged 32 years old from Lamphun province [18].

During these periods (1936–2007), animal infection with echinococcosis was never recorded in Thailand. However, hydatid cysts were reported in slaughtered pigs, cattles, and buffalos in Bangkok and Chiang Mai in the past.

4. Vietnam

Echinococcosis was found in several countries in the Southeast Asian region; however, before 2013, this disease had never been reported to be infected in both animals and humans in Vietnam. The first case of echinococcosis was recorded in a man, aged 42 years, who resides in Thach Thanh district, Thanh Hoa province. This case is also the first indigenous case because he is a farmer who has never traveled abroad. Positive diagnostics are performed by serological tests using ELISA. Patients recovered after treatment with surgery combined with albendazole 800 mg/day for 30 days [5].

The second indigenous case was reported in a woman, aged 48 years, who lived in Phu Yen district, Son La province. She is a medical technician who has never traveled abroad. Positive diagnosis is confirmed by the ELISA test. The observations showed a large number of *Echinococcus* larvae in both lungs, so that no surgery was performed. She then underwent treatment with albendazole 800 mg/day for 30 days. After 12 months, the patient no longer coughed, and only two small cysts remained in her lungs [5]. Based on morphological and molecular methods, *Echinococcus ortleppi* was identified as the source of infection in both of cases. This is the first case of *E. ortleppi* species reported as a cause of echinococcosis in Vietnam and the Southeast Asian region [5, 19].

Previous studies revealed that risk factors for transmission of *E. ortleppi* are more associated with dog and cattle than human. This species was originally described as *E. granulosus* in dogs from South Africa; however, because it develops mostly in cattle as intermediate hosts, *E. ortleppi* is more commonly known as cattle strain (Genotype 5) of *E. granulosus* [32–35]. Currently, it has also been reported to infect others domestic and wild animals, such as buffaloes, sheep, pigs, goats, camels, monkeys, and porcupine [36–40]. In humans, this species has also been reported to have low pathogenicity and be restricted to infect in certain areas. Infection occurs accidentally through ingestion of parasite eggs [6, 41]. Although *E. ortleppi* infection was reported in two indigenous cases from Vietnam, there is no evidence that *E. ortleppi* is a autochthonous disease in northern Vietnam. There are no reports of domestic cattles and dogs infected with this tapeworm species in Vietnam. Most likely, the parasite was introduced from another place through cattle that imported into the country [42].

5. Malaysia

Echinococcosis is very rare in Malaysia. So far, only five cases were reported during more than last five decades. The first human case of pulmonary echinococcosis was reported in a Malay child in 1968. However, there is no detailed information reported during that time. In 1989, a first hepatic hydatidosis was reported in a

59-year-old Indian female. She had complained of fever and right hypochondrial pain for 3 days before inpatient. There was no jaundice. The enlarged liver with span of 17 cm, soft were identified. Ultrasonography examination revealed an encapsulated multiloculated anechoic lesions occurring on the most right of the hepatic lobe. Hydatid cysts and a large cystic lesion were also identified. The patient recovered at 1 year after getting surgical treatment combined with mebendazole 40 mg/kg/day for 30 days postoperatively [32].

The third case was recorded from a 4-year-old girl who was undergoing treatment in a pediatric hospital emergency unit after experiencing repeated cough with high-grade fever, accompanied by severe shortness of breath in 2013. Laboratory investigation was performed with a chest X-ray (CXR) and ultrasound examination. A hypoechoic shadow of a giant cystic lesion and hydatid cyst were detected replacing the whole right lobe of the liver. Surgery was performed, and albendazole was given for 6 months postoperatively. After 1.5 year, the patient demonstrated improved conditions with no recurrence evidence [33].

In 2015, a case of hydatid cyst of the liver was reported in a 55-year-old Chinese-Australian lady. She has migrated from Malaysia to Australia many years ago and works as a nurse assistant. Australia is considered endemic for the disease. There was no history of contact with cattle or dog. This patient presented a long history of abdominal pain, but with no fever or jaundice. She may have experience acute cholangitis, while the hydatid cyst ruptured in the biliary system. The liver cyst showed a calcified wall with only necrotic debris. Laboratory investigation with a chest X-ray, ultrasound examination, and histological analysis strongly suggests patient had chronic hydatid cyst of the liver [34].

The latest record of hydatid hepato-pulmonary fistula caused by *E. granulosus* case was reported in a 58-year-old Malaysian housewife with no history of recent travel outside the country. In the past 3 years, the patient had complained of pain from the right side of the chest and abdominal pain. For the past month before inpatient, she complained severe repetitive attacks of productive cough with yellowish to dark color of sputum and vomiting that was associated with night sweating and fever. Hydatid cysts were identified on top of the right lobe of the liver by using chest X-ray and computerized tomography (CT) of the chest and abdomen. Hydatid patients recovered after getting surgical treatment [35].

6. Philippines

Since 1925, only two local cases of human echinococcosis in the lungs have been reported in the Philippines [43, 44]. No detailed information was reported regarding *Echinococcus* infection in human. In animal, *Echinococcus* cyst was recorded for the first time in a cattle from Los Banos, Laguna, in the 1940s. Echinococcosis in the lungs of a water buffalo and dog were also reported in this country in 1947 [45].

7. Singapore, Cambodia, Lao People's Democratic Republic, Myanmar, and Timor-Leste

In Singapore, Singh et al. reported two imported cases of the disease in 1991 [46]. Echinococcosis has also been observed in humans, cattle, sheep, and pigs in Laos and Cambodia. However, the disease is considered to be very rare in these countries. No information about hydatid disease in Myanmar and Timor-Leste [19, 47].

8. Discussion

A total of 49 cases of echinococcosis was identified in Southeast Asia from 1885 to 2015. Of which, at least 31 case were indigenous, 14 cases were imported, and 4 cases were unknown. The common clinical manifestations found in patients with echinococcosis are swelling or pressure effects from enlarging cysts and pain due to cyst mass [48–51]. However, it is very difficult to estimate the real number of human echinococcosis case in Southeast Asia due to the long asymptomatic period that is usually >5 years [3]. Previous studies in China revealed that echinococcosis manifestations usually appear 2–15 years after infection with nonspecific symptoms [52]. With these possible reasons, the disease may be more prevalent in Southeast Asia; however, they were underdiagnosed.

Most human infections are caused by *E. granulosus* and only two cases with *E. ortleppi*. There was no evidence case with *E. multilocularis* in Southeast Asia. *Echinococcus granulosus* infection is prevalent in areas that association with dogs and livestocks that close contact with dogs [17]. The dog is the definitive host for *E. granulosus* and the main source of human CE worldwide [53]. Livestock, especially sheep and goats, is the most important domestic intermediate host for *E. granulosus*. These worm cysts may also infect other herbivore hosts, e.g., donkeys, buffaloes, pigs, camels, cattle, etc., and are involved in *E. granulosus* transmission [54–56].

Hydatid cysts infection is the most common echinococcosis in this region [3, 5, 17–24, 30, 32, 34, 47, 57–60], while only two cases of alveolar echinococcosis were reported in Thailand [25, 31]. Of all the recorded cases, liver cyst is a leading cause of echinococcosis in Southeast Asia, followed by cyst infection in the lung, peritoneal, kidney, jaw, and foot. Surgical removal and antiparasitic drug therapy have been shown to be beneficial and effective in the management of echinococcosis.

Besides Thailand, the very low incidence was reported in almost all countries in Southeast Asia. The possible reason for the existence of echinococcosis cases might be different in each country. In Indonesia and Malaysia, where the majority of the population is Muslim, this low case might be caused by Muslims not being encouraged to keep dogs. In addition, under-diagnostic and non-reported cases due to the absence of a routine surveillance system for echinococcosis may also contribute to the low incidence in both countries. In Singapore, the low number of cases is likely due to good urban planning with high-quality health standards, so there is very little potential for food-borne parasitic infections in the country [46]. In several other Southeast Asian countries that are epidemiologically similar to Thailand, namely, Cambodia, Myanmar, and Laos, very few reports of echinococcosis cases may be caused by being underdiagnosed and not reported [17]. The same thing is likely to occur in other Southeast Asian countries, such as the Philippines, Vietnam, and Timor-Leste. Although echinococcosis has not been a serious problem for public health in the region, awareness of the disease is needed. The hydatid cyst diagnosis should be inserted in part of the differential diagnosis of all cystic lesion to find out the magnitude of this disease in Southeast Asia [17, 30]. In addition, serological surveys are necessary in each Southeast Asian country to identify the distribution of the disease. Disease surveillance in domestic dogs and livestock is also needed as a prerequisite to understand epidemiological status of echinococcosis in the region.

9. Conclusions

According to this review, the incidence of echinococcosis in Southeast Asia is very low. Thailand is the most prevalent country with echinococcosis in human, followed by very low incidence in Indonesia, Malaysia, Vietnam, the Philippines,

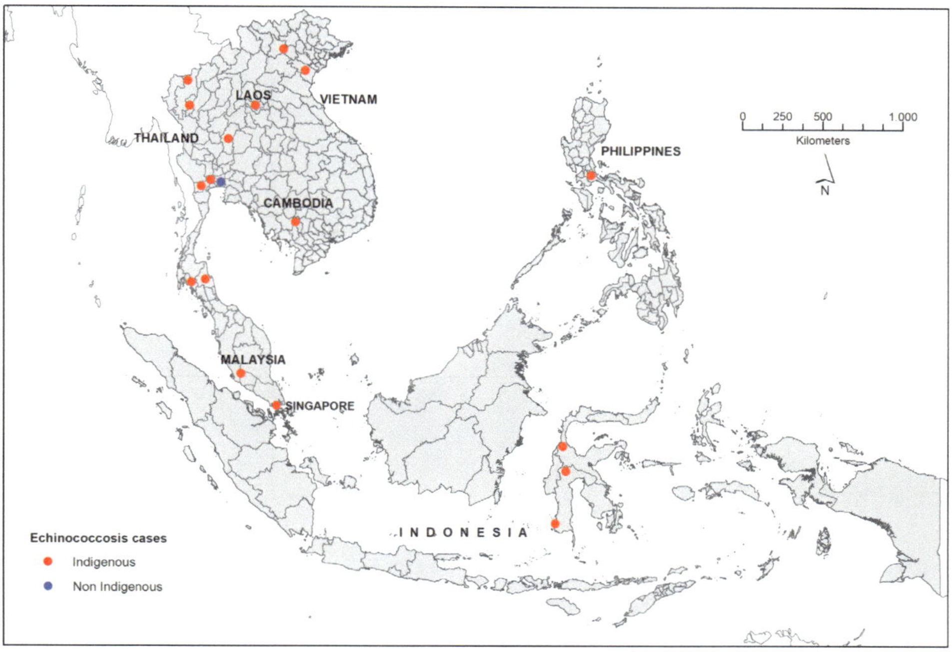

Figure 1.
Map of human cases of echinococcosis distribution in Southeast Asia during 1885–2015. Red dots represent indigenous cases. Blue dots represent nonindigenous cases.

Cambodia, and Lao PDR, and so far there is no report of the disease in Myanmar and Timor-Leste. The disease may be more prevalent; however, there were underdiagnosed and not reported. Disease surveillance in human, domestic dogs, and livestock are necessary in Southeast Asian countries to identify the distribution of the disease. In addition, awareness and strengthening diagnosis for the disease are also needed in part of *Echinococcus* surveillance to identify the real incidence and magnitude in this region (**Figure 1**).

Acknowledgements

The authors would like to thank all of the data contributor for echinococcosis in all countries in Southeast Asia.

Conflict of interest

The authors declare no conflict of interest.

Abbreviations

G	genotype
AE	alveolar echinococcosis
CE	cystic echinococcosis
CT	computerized tomography
CXR	chest x-ray
ELISA	enzyme-linked immunosorbent assay

Author details

Triwibowo Ambar Garjito[1*], Mujiyanto Mujiyanto[1] and Mohammad Sudomo[2]

1 Institute for Vector and Reservoir Control Research and Development, National Institute of Health Research and Development, Ministry of Health Indonesia, Indonesia

2 National Institute of Health Research and Development, Ministry of Health Indonesia, Indonesia

*Address all correspondence to: triwibowo@litbang.depkes.go.id

References

[1] Wen H, Vuitton L, Tuxun T, et al. Echinococcosis: Advances in the 21st century. Clinical Microbiology Reviews. 2019;**32**:1-39

[2] Mcmanus DP, Zhang W, Li J, et al. Echinococcosis. Lancet. 2003;**362**: 1295-1304

[3] DP MM. Echinococcosis with Particular Reference to Southeast Asia. 1st ed. Elsevier Ltd.; 2010

[4] Nakao M, Lavikainen A, Yanagida T, et al. Phylogenetic systematics of the genus Echinococcus (Cestoda: Taeniidae). International Journal for Parasitology. 2013;**43**:1017-1020

[5] De Nguyen V, Le Van D. The first report of two cases of cystic echinococcosis in the lung by Echinococcus ortleppi infection, in Vietnam. Research and Reports in Tropical Medicine. 2017;**8**:45-51

[6] Balbinotti H, Santos G, Badaraco J, et al. Echinococcus ortleppi (G5) and echinococcus granulosus sensu sticto (G1) loads in cattle from Southern Brazil. Veterinary Parasitology. 2012; **188**:255-260

[7] Van Der E. Echinococcus blass ult de lever (Hydatid cyst from the liver). Geneesk. Tijdschr. Ned.-Indie;**24**

[8] Boerma V, Kiewiet D, Verspijck M. Echinococcus infectie (Echinococcus infection). Geneesk. Tijdschr. Ned.-Indie. 1921;**61**:111-112

[9] Snijders E. Een merkwaardige lever patient (An extraordinary liver patient). Geneesk. Tijdschr. Ned.-Indie. 1939;**79**: 2485

[10] Amran A, Gella M, Abadi K. Kista hidatid pada hati: laporan kasus (A Hydatid Cyst in the Liver: A Case Report). Jakarta: Kongres Nasional IKARI; 1988

[11] Abadi K, Jobs S, Gella M, et al. Kasus penyakit hidatid unikuler di Ujung Pandang, Sulawesi Selatan (A Unilocular Hydatidosis Case in Ujung Panjang, South Sulawesi). Bogor: National Parasitology Seminar and Fourth P4I Congress; 1988

[12] Vrijburg A. Uit de praktijk in Deli (from a practice in Deli). Ned-Indisch Bl Diergeneesk. 1907;**19**:217

[13] Smit H. Echinococcosis in Nederlandsch-Indie (Echinococcosis in Netherlands-Indies). Ned-Indisch Bl Diergeneesk. 1920;**32**:25

[14] Muller H, Fooy J. Echinococcose bij het varken in Nederlandsch-Indie (Echinococcosis in pigs in Netherlands-Indies). Ned-Indisch Bl Diergeneesk. 1929;**41**:466

[15] Kranefeld F, Douwes J. Aanvullende lijst van voor Nederlandsch-Indie nieuwe parsitaire wormen bij zoogdieren en vogels. Ned-Indisch Bl Diergeneesk. 1940;**52**:178-180

[16] Carney W, Cross J, Wheeling C, et al. Natural infection of Echinococcus granulosus in dogs from Sulawesi, Indonesia. Southeast Asian Journal of Tropical Medicine and Public Health. 1974;**5**:385-389

[17] Wiwanitki V. A summary of hydatid disease in Thailand. The Internet Journal of Tropical Medicine. 2004;**2**:1-5

[18] Waikagul J, Dekumyoy P, Anantaphruti MT. Taeniasis, cycticercosis and echinococcosis in Thailand. Parasitology International. 2006;**55**:175-180

[19] Morakote N, Thamprasert K, Lojanapiwat B, et al. Cystic

echinococcosis in Thailand with a species note on detection by serology in one family. The Southeast Asian Journal of Tropical Medicine and Public Health. 2007;**38**:796-799

[20] Chitrapatima K, Muntarbhorn S. Hydatid cysts in the lung treated by total pneumonectomy. Journal of the Medical Association of Thailand. 1952; **35**:1-7

[21] Koanantakool T, Subbannachart P, Tengtrisorn C, et al. The first pulmonary hydatid cyst in Central Cest Hospital. Journal of Communicable Diseases. 1991;**17**:178-184

[22] Thanakitcharu S, Saenghirunvattana S, Tovaranonte P, et al. Pulmonary hydatid disease: a case report. Thai Journal of Tuberculosis Chest Diseases. 1992;**13**:245-251

[23] Leelakusolwong S. Surgery of hydatid cyst of the liver. Thai Journal of Gastroenterology. 1995;**3**:49-53

[24] Leungsuwan P. Hydatid cyst of liver. Siriraj Hospital Gazette. 1960;**12**: 797-800

[25] Kheedler W. Some rare diseases of Siam Echinococcus cyst. Journal of the Medical Association of Thailand. 1936; **19**:773-781

[26] Na-songkla S. Echinococcal cyst of lung: the first indigenous case. In: Scientific meeting of tropical medicine, Faculty of Tropical Medicine. 1980

[27] Rangkasem K, Kattipatanapong W, Thadadoltip W, et al. Human echinococcosis: report of two cases of the hydatid disease at the lungs and liver. Chiang Mai Medical Bulletin. 1995; **35**:28-29

[28] Vatanatumrak B, Manothaya C, Udomchanya S. Hydatid cyst of the lung: a case report. The Thai Journal of Surgery. 1980;**1**:118-120

[29] Thamprasert K. Renal hydatid cyst (echinococcosis) in Maharaj Nakorn Chiang Mai Hospital: a case report and review of literature. Chiang Mai Medical Bulletin. 1993;**32**:31-35

[30] Riengchan P, Suankatay C, Wilde H, et al. Hydatid disease of the liver: the first indigenous case in Thailand and review of the literature. Journal of the Medical Association of Thailand. 2004;**87**:725-729

[31] Limawongpranee S, Suankratay C, Wilde H, et al. Alveolar echinococcosis: an unusual liver mass in a Thai patient. Journal of the Medical Association of Thailand. 2004;**56**:308-314

[32] Jalleh R, Nuruddin R, Krishnan M. Hydatidosis: diagnostic and therapeutic aspects. Singapore Medical Journal. 1989;**30**:210-212

[33] Moshin A, Khorsheed M. Massive hydatid cyst in four years old child patient; Case report. Journal of Advances in Medicine and Medical Research. 2013;**3**:31-35

[34] Hayati MPS, Eugene CBT, Jin BJ, et al. Chronic hydatid cyst in Malaysia: a rare occurrence. Malaysian Journal of Medical Sciences. 2015;**22**:79-83

[35] Ali TI. Ibrahim OEm, Al-sultan II. Hydatid hepatic-broncho-pleural (hepato-pulmonary) fistula caused by Echinococcosis granulosa: a zoonotic case report. Malaysian Journal of Veterinary Research. 2018;**9**: 91-97

[36] Boufana B, Stidworthy M, Bell S, Chantrey J, Masters N, Unwin S, et al. Echinococcus and Taenia spp. from captive mammals in the United Kingdom. Veterinary Parasitology. 2012;**190**:95-103

[37] Amer S, Helal I, Kamau E, Feng Y, Xiao L. Molecular characterization of Echinococcus granulosus sensu lato

from farm animals in Egypt. PLOS One. 2015;**10**:e0118509

[38] Pednekar R, Gatne M, Thompson R, Traub R. Molecular and morphological characterization of Echinococcus from food producing animals in India. Veterinary Parasitology. 2009;**165**:58-65

[39] Dinkel A, Njoroge E, Zimmermann A, Walz M, Zeyhle E, Elmahdi I, et al. A PCR system for detection of species and genotypes of the Echinococcus granulosus-complex, with reference to the epidemiological situation in Eastern Africa. International Journal for Parasitology. 2004;**34**: 645-653

[40] Mbaya H, Magambo J, Njenga S, Zeyhle E, Mbae C, Mulinge E, et al. Echinococcus spp. in Central Kenya: a different story. Parasitology Research. 2014;**113**:3789-3794

[41] Rojas CA, Romig T, Lighttowlers M. Echinococcus granulosus sensu lato genotypes infecting humans-review of current knowledge. International Journal for Parasitology. 2014;**44**:9-18

[42] Deplazes P, Rinaldi L, Rojas C, Torgerson P, Harandi M, Romig T, et al. Global distribution of Alveolar and Cystic Echinococcosis. Advances in Parasitology. 2017;**95**:315-493

[43] De Leon W, Leiva L. Echinococcus cyst of the human lung. The Philippine Journal of Science. 1925;**27**:361-370

[44] Lavadia P, Canlas B, Durban V. Hydatid cyst of the lung (a case report in a Filipino). Journal of the Philippine Medical Association. 1960;**36**:702-708

[45] Tubangui MA. A summary of the parasitic worms reported from the Philippines. The Philippine Journal of Science. 1947;**76**:225-322

[46] Singh M, Hian Y, Lay-Hoon C. Current status of food-borne parasitic zoonoses in Singapore. The Southeast Asian Journal of Tropical Medicine and Public Health. 1991;**22**:27-35

[47] Matossian R, Rickard M, Smyth J. Hydatidosis: a global problem of increasing importance. Bulletin of the World Health Organization. 1977;**55**: 499-507

[48] Ammann R, Eckert J. Cestodes: Echinococcus Gastroenterol. Clinics of North America. 1996;**25**:655-689

[49] Schaefer J, Khan M. Echinococcosis (hydatid disease): lessons from experience with 59 patients. Reviews of Infectious Diseases. 1991;**13**:243-247

[50] Kammerer W, Schantz P. Echinococcal disease. Infectious Disease Clinics of North America. 1993;**7**: 605-618

[51] Lewis J, Koss N, Kerstein M. A review of echinococcal disease. Annals of Surgery. 1975;**181**:390-396

[52] Craig PS. Epidemiology of echinococcosis in western China. In: Torgerson P, Shaikenov B, editors. Echinococcosis in Central Asia: Problems and Solutions. Zürich, Dauir; 2004. pp. 43-58

[53] Carmena D, Cardona G. Canine echinococcosis: Global epidemiology and genotype diversity. Acta Tropica. 2013;**128**:441-460

[54] Eckert J, Deplazes P, Craig PS, Gemmell MA, Gottstein B, Health D, et al. Echinococcosis in animals: clinical aspects, diagnosis and treatment. In: Eckert J, Gemmell MA, Meslin FX, Pawlowski ZS, editors. WHO/OIE Manual on Echinococcosis in Humans and Animals: A Public Health Problem of Global Concern. Paris, France: WHO/ OIE; 2001

[55] Jenkins DJ. *Echinococcus granulosus* in Australia, widespread and doing well.

International Journal for Parasitology. 2006;**55**:203-206

[56] Boufana B, Lahmar S, Rebai W, Safta ZB, Jebali L, Ammar A, et al. Genetic variability and haplotypes of Echinococcus isolates from Tunisia. Transactions of the Royal Society of Tropical Medicine and Hygiene. 2014; **18**:706-714

[57] Romig T, Ebi D, Wassermann M. Taxonomy and molecular epidemiology of Echinococcus granulosus sensu lato. Veterinary Parasitology. 2015;**213**:76-84

[58] Ortlepp J. Echinococcus in dogs from Pretoria and vicinity. The Onderstepoort Journal of Veterinary Science and Animal Industry. 1934;**3**(1): 97-108

[59] Thompson R, McManus D. Towards a taxonomic revision of the genus Echinococcus. Trends in Parasitology. 2002;**18**:452-457

[60] Shi Y, Wan X, Wang Z, Li J, Jiang Z, Yang Y. First description of Echinococcus ortleppi infection in China. Parasites & Vectors. 2019;**12**:398

Section 3

Parasitology

Chapter 3

Taenia solium Cysticercosis in Pigs and Human: A Review of Epidemiological Data in West Africa (1990–2019)

Rebecca Weka, Pam Luka, Ndudim Ogo and Paul Weka

Abstract

Taenia solium taeniasis/cysticercosis/neurocysticercosis is a neglected zoonotic disease endemic in sub-Saharan Africa, Latin-American and Asia and is an emerging public health and economic problem. The association between cysticercosis and epilepsy has been documented worldwide including West Africa. Poor sanitary conditions, traditional pig farming and poverty play an important role in perpetuation of *Taenia solium*. There has been limited research undertaken in *T. solium* in human and pigs in some West African countries, where prevalence of taeniasis was up 40%, human cysticercosis 10.3%, porcine cysticercosis 32.5–39.6% and epilepsy 28.0/1000–43.0/1000. The study identified porcine cysticercosis in 18 countries, human cysticercosis in 19 countries, taeniasis in 4 countries and epilepsy was reported in 25 countries. The aim of this study is to review scientific literature on the epidemiology of *T. solium* infections in pigs and humans in Western Africa and document data on the prevalence of epilepsy in the region. The objective is to document occurrence of disease in West Africa so as to offer options available for control. The study conducted literature search of online international databases of published resources for information on *T. solium* in Western Africa and Epilepsy from 1990 to 2018.

Keywords: *Taenia solium*, epilepsy, human, pigs, West Africa, literature search, epidemiology

1. Introduction

Parasitic zoonoses are becoming increasingly important in the spectrum of emerging and re-emergent diseases for both developed and developing countries, and are typically associated with poor marginalized countries in low-income countries. They are regarded as disease of the poorest among the poor [1–3]. *Taenia solium* is found in sub-Saharan Africa, Central Asia and Latin America where domestic pig husbandry is practiced, poverty, illiteracy and deficient sanitary infrastructures are common [1, 4, 5]. Similarly, the disease has been reported in urban areas where most of the infected pigs are transported and consumed. The incidence of the disease in humans is increasing and now is a re-emerging disease in some developed countries and in areas of non-endemicity, due to international travel and immigration [6, 7]. Hence cysticercosis/neurocysticercosis/teaniosis complex caused by the larval stage of *T. solium* in both pigs and humans remains a significant cause of human morbidity and mortality in many parts of the world. It is seriously affecting pig production and also considered as a public health and economic problem in many developing countries affecting food security and negatively impacts the nutritional and economic well-being of the small holder farming community [8, 9].

2. Life cycle

2.1 Life cycle and pathogenesis

Taenia solium life cycle is sustained where free roaming pigs, have access to contaminated feces of tapeworm carriers. *T. solium* has a complex two host life cycle and is cyclically transmitted between pigs and man. Humans are the only definitive host and harbor the adult stages of these cestodes following ingestion of insufficiently cooked pork meat infested with cysticerci. Infection with the adult stage is relatively innocuous and carries mild clinical manifestations leading to taeniasis [1–11]. Pigs are the natural intermediate host, while human's acts as the accidental dead-end intermediate host and are both infected with *T. solium* by ingestion of embryonated eggs from feces of tapeworm carriers from contaminated soil, water, vegetation/foods to form cysticerci. Infection with the cysticerci leads to more severe symptoms including headache and neurocysticercosis when the pathology occurs in the CNS [11].

2.2 Epidemiology

Neurocysticercosis has been considered to be the most common parasitic infestation of the central nervous system and the single most common cause of preventable acquired epilepsy and mortality in developing countries [12–14], and a strong correlation was reported between the prevalence of epilepsy and seropositivity against *T. solium* cysticercosis [15]. The association between cysticercosis and epilepsy has been documented as a leading neurological condition worldwide including West Africa. Epilepsy is a frequent chronic neurologic disorder that affects approximately 70 million people of all ages worldwide [15] Studies of [10] in 2010 reported that the median prevalence of active epilepsy was 4.9/1000 (2.3–10.3) for developed countries, 12.7/1000 (3.5–45.5) and 5.9/1000 (3.4–10.2) in rural and urban studies in developing countries. Neurocysticercosis has been associated with 30% of adult onset epilepsy in endemic regions where 10–20% of the general population can have brain lesions consistent with neurocysticercosis on CT scans [16]. Neurocysticercosis creates a tremendous economic burden in endemic areas incurring significant costs due to diagnosis, treatment and disability [17]. Poor sanitary conditions, traditional pig farming, lack of awareness of the disease and poverty play an important role in the perpetuation of the *Taenia solium*/cysticercosis, and are present in West Africa [18]. Research in the region on *Taenia solium* cysticercosis and taeniasis in both human and pigs has been limited. Prevalence information of the disease in some countries within the region has been scanty leading to underestimation of the prevalence, epidemiology and clinical impacts of the disease which has made it difficult to make definitive recommendations on control strategies. Data on porcine and human cysticercosis are available from several countries. However, there is no recent information on *T. solium* taeniasis-cysticercosis complex in some countries including Guinea Bissau, Liberia, Ivory coast and Sierra-Leone [19] as shown in **Tables 1** and **2**. The aim of this study is to review scientific and gray literature and to identify the empirical data on *T. solium* taeniasis/human/porcine cysticercosis/neurocysticercosis/epilepsy in West Africa and the risk factors responsible for the epidemiology of *T. solium* cysticercosis in order to understand the differences in exposure to the parasite in endemic areas around the world. This will give an update and compile the current knowledge on *T. solium* in Western Africa, including risk factors for infections in pigs and humans

Author	Country/location	Diagnosis	Total	Prevalence	Type of study
[20]	Benin, Southern Benin	Meat inspection	118.073	0.06–0.69%	Abattoir
[21]	Burkina Faso, Ouagadougou	Meat inspection	62,311	0.22 (n = 139)	Abattoir
[22]	Burkina Faso	B158/B60 Ag-ELISA	336	32.5–39.6%	Cross sectional
[58]	Burkina Faso	Meat inspection	117,026	0.57% (n = 673)	Abattoir
[59]	Ghana, Kumasi	Ante mortem/post mortem	4121	2.31% (n = 95)	Cross sectional
[60]	Ghana, Upper East Region	Post mortem	60	11.70%	Cross sectional
[61]	Nigeria, Bodija, Ibadan, Oyo State	Meat inspection	593	1.01% (n = 6)	Abattoir
[62]	Nigeria, Michika, Adamawa State,	Post mortem	247	3.2% (n = 8)	Cross sectional
[65]	Nigeria, Nasarawa and Gonin Gora,Chikun, Kaduna	Post mortem	43	9.3% (n = 4)	Cross sectional
[63]	Nigeria, Jalingo, Taraba State	Post mortem	323	4.95% (n = 16)	Cross sectional
[23]	Nigeria, Zuru, Kebbi State	Lingual, post mortem	4208	5.85% (n = 205) 14.4% (n = 118)	Cross sectional
[64]	Nigeria, Bodija, Ibadan,	Post mortem	250	4.4% (n = 11)	Cross sectional
[24]	Nigeria, Ibi Taraba State	Antemortem/post mortem	4380	6.25% (n = 274)	Cross sectional
[25]	Nigeria, Nsukka Enugu State	Lingual/post mortem	2358	20% (n = 483)	Cross sectional
[26]	Nigeria, Enugu State Udenu, Igbo-Eze South Nsukka Enugu State	Post mortem	379	2.4% (n = 9)	Cross sectional
[66]	Nigeria, Jos	Antibody ELISA	115	46% (n = 29)	Cross sectional
[67]	Gambia, Western region	Lingual, Ag-ELISA	1705	4.8%	Cross sectional
[67]	Senegal	Lingual, Ag-ELISA	1705	6.4–13.2%	Cross sectional

Table 1.
Selected studies of porcine cysticercosis in West Africa 1980–2019.

Author	Country/location	Diagnosis	Total	Epilepsy (n)	Neurocysticercosis	Cysticercosis	Taeniasis
[27]	Benin	Capture recapture/Neurlogist	3134	20.1/1000 (n = 66) GP	ND	ND	ND
[28]	Benin	Capture recapture/Neurlogist	11,668	12.7/1000 (148) GP	ND	ND	ND
[29]	Benin, Savolou	Ab-ELISA, skull/muscle X-ray and pathol. of cysts	1443	1.5 (22/1443), 17/186 GP	4.0% (n = 57)	1% (n = 14 skin nodules)	ND
[29]	Benin, Vekky	Ab-ELISA, skull/muscle X-ray and pathol. of cysts	319	GP	3.5% (319)	ND	ND
[29]	Benin	Ab-ELISA, skull/muscle X-ray and pathol. of cysts	2625	GP	1.6% (n = 41)	ND	ND
[30]	Benin	AB,ELISA/(EITB)	2625	41/1.3% (35) GP	ND	ND	ND
[31]	Benin	Questionnaire,clinical/neurologist	13,046	8.05/1000 (n = 105), GP	ND	ND	ND
[32]	Burkina Faso	B158/B60 AG-ELISA	3609	GP	ND	0–11.5% (n = 120)	ND
[33]	Burkina Faso	Ag B158/B60 ELISA	1729/1719	GP	ND	3·8% (n = 65) CC 2.7% (n = 47) (2.7%)	ND
[34]	Burkina Faso´ a	B158/B60 Ag-ELISA	763	GP	ND	6.29% (n = 48)	ND
[35]	Burkina Faso	B158/B60 Ag-ELISA questionnaire/neurologist	3696	3.9% (n = 145), GP		3.4% (n = 129)	ND
[36]	Burkina Faso	AgELISA/CT scan/neurologist	888	4.4$(39) epi, VLVL	29% (20/68)	ND	ND
[37]	Burkina Faso	Ag-ELISA, physician	888	4.5% (39) of 70 VL	5/39 epileptics (12.8%), 3.4% (28/814)	ND	ND
[34]	Burkina Faso	Questionnaire neurologist	4768	669 (14.0%), VL	0.6% (29)	ND	ND
[38]	Burkina-Faso		16,627	10.6 per 1000, CB	ND	ND	ND
[39]	Ghana Bunkpuru	Kato-Katz technique	494		ND	ND	13.15% (n = 65)

Author	Country/location	Diagnosis	Total	Epilepsy (*n*)	Neurocysticercosis	Cysticercosis	Taeniasis
[40]	GhanaKintampo	Questionnairesclinicians/western blot	586,607	10.1/1000	ND	0.01	ND
[41]	Senegal	Direct fecal examination		ND	ND	ND	2/43* 4.65
[42]		Fecal egg count		ND	ND	ND	4/43** 9.30
[42]		Worm expulsion/amorphological identification	ND	ND	ND	ND	1/43***2.33
[43]	Nigeria ebonyi/ benue state	Questionnaire	2500 and 6000	(n = 52) 20.8/1000 and (28) 4.7/1000, PB	ND	ND	ND
[44]	Nigeria Agu-Abor/ Enugu	Questionnaire, medical	8228	0.6%/1000 (n = 49)	ND	ND	ND
[48]	Nigeria Kaduna	Ab-ELISA	300			14.3% (n = 43)	ND
[45]	Nigeria Abuja	An 8000 B-Scan Scanmate				Ocular cysticercosis	
[70]	Nigeria Ukpo,Dunukofia Anambra state,	Door to door Questionnaire, neurologist	6800	4.3/1000 (n = 29)	ND	ND	ND
[46]	Nigeria Odeda, Ogun State,	Sodium acetate acetic acid formalin concentration method (SAF-Ether)	428		ND		40% (n = 175)
[25]	Nigeria Nsukka Enugu State,	Stool microscopy	1525		ND	ND	8·6% (n = 131)
[47]	Nigeria Jos	Ab-ELISA	125		ND	9.6% (n = 12)	ND
[48]	Nigeria Nasarawa	Copro Ag ELISA, questionnaire	10				30 (n = 3)
[49]	Nigeria Ile-Ife	Surgeon/histopathological, biopsy				Cysticercosis of breast	ND

Author	Country/location	Diagnosis	Total	Epilepsy (n)	Neurocysticercosis	Cysticercosis	Taeniasis
[50]	Nigeria, Edo State,	Surgeon, histopathological				Cysticercosis in the anterior chamber	ND
[51]	Nigeria	Questionnaire	18,951	5.3/1000 101, CB			ND
[71]	Nigeria Osun	Surgery, Occular Ultrasound				Intraocular cysticercosis	ND
[42]	Senegal Soutou	(Ag-ELISA) and (EITB),CT scan	403		7.69 (n = 31)/7.69 (n = 31)	23.3 (10/43)	ND
[52]	Senegal Pikine, Dakar	Questionnaire, physician, electroencephalography	4500	(n = 64) 14.2/1000	ND	ND	ND
[53]	Senegal		7682	8.3/per 1000	ND	ND	ND
[41]	Liberia		4436	(123) 28.0per 1000			
[54]	Liberia		2733	43.0 per 1000, CB	ND	ND	ND
[55]	Mauritania	Neurologist	236	34.7% (n = 82), HB			
[56]	Togo, Tone		9155 for epi and 1343 for cyst (n = 5264) 2.4%	18.6%/1000, GB	ND	38/1000	ND
[57]	Togo, the Kozah district of North Togo		5264	(n = 88) 16/1000	ND	23.3% (n = 123)	ND

2/43 4.65, foot note =direct microscopy.*
*4/43** 9.30, foot note = Ritchie formol ether method.*
*1/43*** 2.33,foot note= Worm expulsion.*

Table 2.
Selected prevalence of human cysticersosis and epilepsy in west African countries.

cysticercosis (HCC) from endemic communities. The objective of the study will be to review and document data on the prevalence of human cysticercosis/neurocysticercosis in the region with emphasis on epilepsy.

2.3 Methods

A systematic literature search was done on studies carried out on cysticercosis in humans and pigs, seroprevalence of cysticercosis in humans and pigs, neurocysticercosis/taeniasis, risk factors for transmission of cysticercosis and epilepsy in West Africa published between 1980 and 2019. This search focused on the articles in which data was obtained using the following techniques and protocols: (1) enzyme-linked immunoelectrotransfer blot (EITB), (2) enzyme-linked immunosorbent assay (B158/B60 Ag-ELISA or HP10 Ag-ELISA), (3) copro-antigen ELISA and real-time polymerase chain reaction assay (copro-PCR). Language restriction was applied, the considered languages were English and French. The selected databases for this study were: PubMed (http://www.ncbi.nlm.nih.gov/pubmed/), Google scholar and others. The search was performed from May 22 to August 22, 2019.

2.4 Literature search

The following data were included in this study (1) peer-reviewed studies of *T. solium* taeniasis/cysticercosis/neurocysticercosis, porcine cysticercosis and epilepsy in West Africa. (2) "Gray literature" on *T. solium* taeniasis/cysticercosis, neurocysticercosis presence in West Africa which consisted of informally published written materials including reports. We performed a literature search using PubMed (http://www.ncbi.nlm.nih.gov/pubmed/) with date restriction from January 1, 1980 to January 5, 2019 using the following search term: (solium OR Tapeworm OR Taeniasis OR Taeni* OR Taeniosis OR Neurocysticercosis OR Cysticerc* OR epilepsy) AND West Africa (Benin OR Burkina Faso OR Ivory Coast OR Cape Verde OR Gambia OR Ghana OR Guinea OR Guinea Bissau OR Liberia OR Libya OR Malawi OR Mali OR Mauritania OR Niger OR Nigeria OR Senegal OR Sierra Leone OR Togo). We also searched other databases such as Google Scholar (http://scholar.google.com), Cab Direct (http://www.cab direct.org) and African Journals Online (http://www.ajol.info) using the following keywords: "*Taenia solium*," "porcine cysticercosis," "neurocysticercosis," "human cysticercosis" and "taeniasis" Epilepsy, West Africa.

2.5 Data extraction and collection

Presence of *T. solium* in this study was defined as a documented case of disease related to the tapeworm, whether it was diagnosed and documented as human cysticercosis, neurocysticercosis, porcine cysticercosis, taeniasis or epilepsy. Initially, we reviewed all titles and abstracts, if accessible, and excluded studies outside West Africa, and studies with no specified diagnostic technique, studies written in languages other than English and French, and studies not having full paper, that is, abstracts only experimental studies were also excluded.

2.6 Study selection

Figure 1 describes the review process and the number of articles selected at each stage of the review. From an initial number of 550 articles, only 121 were eventually used. The search selected by removal of duplicate studies from the title selection and studies performed before 1980. Secondly, another set of articles were excluded due to: (1) parasites other than *T. solium*; (2) studies performed in non-west African

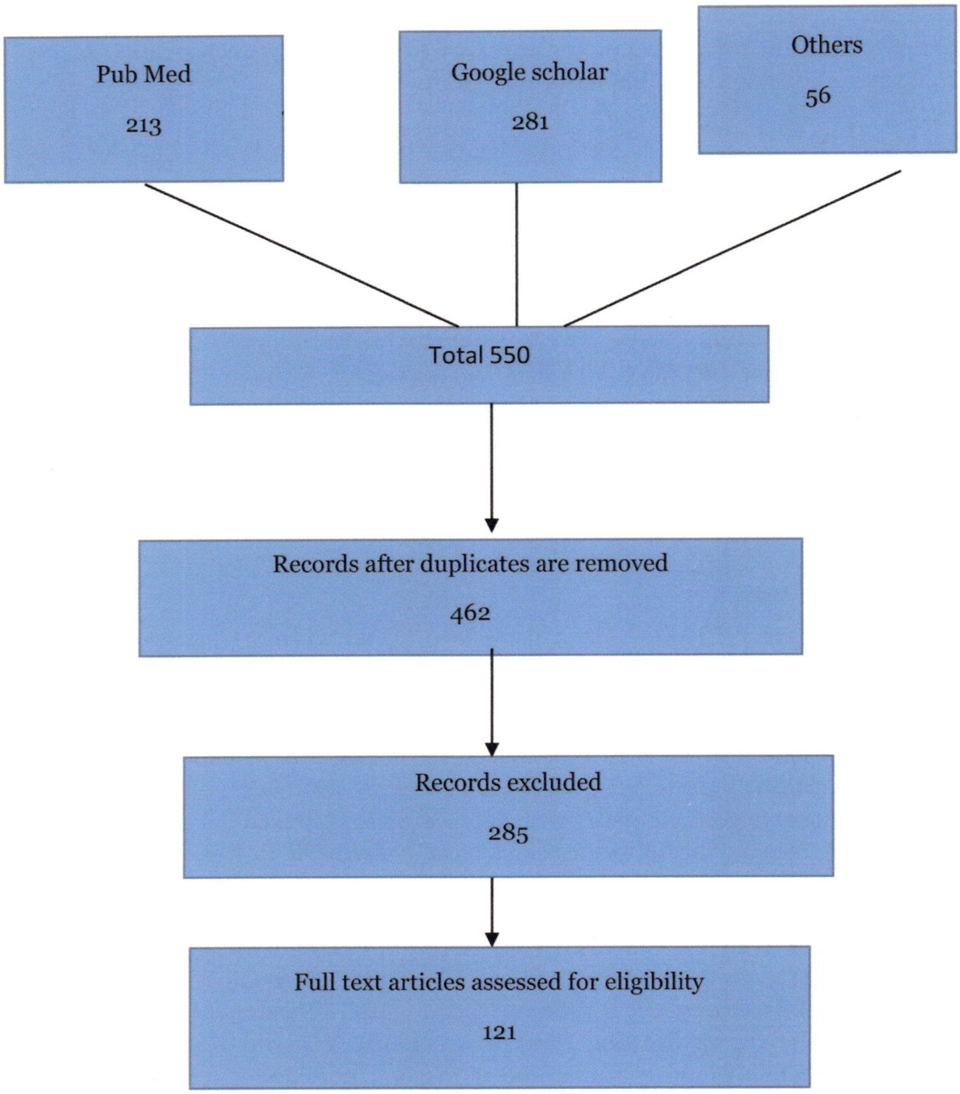

Figure 1.
Flow diagram.

countries; (3) articles written in languages other than French and English; (4) studies not presenting original data and/or the techniques and protocols performed on their studies and (5) studies not related to *T. solium* epidemiology and epilepsy in West African countries. Finally, when full texts were read, the following were selected. Community-based studies, case reports, HCC prevalence reports available, HCC diagnosis using the EITB and Ag ELISA, porcine cysticercosis using carcass inspection and Ab and Ag ELISA, Taeniasis studies based on Copro-Ag ELISA and stool microscopy, and epilepsy studies based on questionnaire, medical or non-medical sources.

3. Results

The search identified 66 studies that reported the prevalence of *T. solium* taeniasis/cysticercosis/neurocysticercosis and epilepsy in West Africa from 1980 to 2019.The study identified porcine cysticercosis in 18 countries, human cysticercosis in 19 countries, taeniasis in 4 countries and epilepsy was reported in 25 countries

(**Tables 1** and **2**). **Figure 1** shows the flow chart of the selection of literature for the informed prevalence estimations of studies included in this review; 8 from Benin (1PC/7HCC/PWE), 11 from Burkina Faso (3PC/8HCC/PWE), 1 from Gambia (PC), 4 from Ghana (2PC/1EP/1TE), 2 from Liberia (PWE), 1 from Mali (PWE), 1 from Mauritania (PWE), 24 from Nigeria (PC10/HCC/PWE14), 3 from Senegal (1PC/2PWEI) and 4 from Togo (4 PWE).

3.1 Porcine cysticercosis in West Africa

One epidemiological studies from Benin [20] used carcass inspection to determine the prevalence of porcine inspection and obtained a prevalence of 0.06–0.69% among a total of 118,073, slaughtered pigs. Two studies from Burkina Faso used carcass inspection to determine the prevalence of porcine cysticercosis and obtained a prevalence of 0.22–0.57% in a total of 179,337 pigs [21, 58]. One study used B158/B60 Ag-ELISA to determine the prevalence of active cysticercosis in pigs and obtained a seroprevalence of 32.5–39.6% among 336 pigs [22]. Two studies from Ghana determined the prevalence of porcine cysticercosis by carcass inspection and obtained the prevalence of 2.31–11.70% [59, 60], among a total of 4181 pigs. A total of 10 studies in Nigeria determined the prevalence of porcine cysticercosis by carcass inspection and obtained a prevalence of 1–20% [23–26, 61–65] among a total population of 12,781 pigs. While one study determined the seroprevalence of porcine cysticercosis and obtained a seroprevalence of 46% IgG antibodies among 115 pigs [66]. A study in Senegal determined the prevalence of porcine cysticercosis by lingual inspection and obtained a prevalence of 0.1–1.0%, while Ag-ELISA gave a seroprevalence of 4.8% [67]. All the data are presented in **Table 1**.

3.2 Human cysticercosis, taeniasis and epilepsy in West Africa

Sero-epidemiological studies from 16 countries were selected for the West African region, 3 studies [29] from Benin used Ab-ELISA, skull/muscle X-ray and pathology of cysts and a study used both Ab-ELISA and EITB [30]. The total number of individuals sampled for serological testing in this region was 4387. Prevalence of circulating antibodies ranged from 1 to 4%. Detailed description of each study is given in **Table 2**. The total number of individuals examined for epilepsy survey in the region was 27,848, excluding 1443 individuals that were involved in the serological study by [29]. Three studies used door-to-door method of survey in estimating the prevalence of epilepsy [27, 30, 31]. Two of the authors used capture/recapture method. They used questionnaires/neurologist to diagnose epileptics [27, 30, 31] and according to definition by the ILAE 1989, and PAANS [68, 69]. The prevalence of epilepsy in the country ranged from 8.08/1000 to 20.1/1000. A study [29] linked the 1.5% seroprevalence epilepsy to the prevalence of human cysticercosis. A 0–29% human cysticercosis seroprevalence in Burkina Faso was obtained from six studies using Ag-ELISA [32–34, 36, 37] and the prevalence of epilepsy in the region ranged from 4.5 to 14% per 1000. The total individuals sampled for seroprevalence studies were 13,413. Three of the studies associated the prevalence of epilepsy to cysticercosis [36, 37]. Two studies [34, 38] estimated the prevalence of epilepsy only, with a total individuals sample size of 29,315 excluding studies that associated the prevalence of epilepsy with cysticercosis.

Human taeniasis from Ghana was obtained from a study performing the Katao Khazt method and obtained a prevalence of 13.3% in a total sample size of 44 individuals [39]. Human cysticercosis in Ghana was obtained from a study by western blot and obtained a prevalence of 0.01% and the same study estimated the prevalence of epilepsy as 10.1/1000 in a total population size of 586,607 [40].

Human cysticercosis from Nigeria was obtained from two studies [47, 48] by using Ab ELISA with prevalence of cysticercosis ranging from 9.6 to 14.3% in a total of 425 individuals. There were five studies selected for epilepsy [43, 44, 51, 70] with prevalence ranging from 4.3/1000 to 20.8/1000 in a total of 64,979 individuals for the epilepsy study. Five studies in the region were case report of cysticercosis [45, 49, 50, 71] involving the ocular and breast cysticercosis. Human taeniasis was obtained from two studies by stool microscopy [25, 46] with a prevalence ranging from 8.6 to 40% among a total of 1953 individuals in the region. Human cysticercosis in Senegal was obtained from one study performing antigen and antibody ELISA [42]. The total number of individuals in the study were 403, and prevalence of both antigen and antibody was 7.6%.The prevalence of epilepsy in the country was obtained from two selected studies [52, 53] and the prevalence of epilepsy ranged from 8.3/1000 to 14.2/1000 in a total of 12,182 individuals. Prevalence of epilepsy from Liberia was obtained from two studies [41, 54] and the prevalence of epilepsy across the region ranged from 28.0/1000 to 43.0/1000 among a total of 7169. Prevalence of epilepsy from Mauritania was obtained in one study [55] with a prevalence of 34.7/1000 in a total of 236 individuals. Human cysticercosis was obtained from two sero-epidemiological studies from Togo by antibody ELISA and gave a prevalence of 23.3 [57] and cysticercosis 38/1000 [56] among a total of 14,419 individuals. The two studies also estimated the prevalence of epilepsy and obtained 16/1000 and 18.6/1000 [56, 57] among a total of 6607. A detailed description of each study is given in **Table 2**.

3.3 Risk factors for human cysticercosis in West Africa

Out of the selected articles reviewed, 16 identified risk factors associated with the prevalence of *Taenia solium* cysticercosis, taeniasis, epilepsy and porcine cysticercosis. Lack of proper meat inspection, clandestine slaughtering of pigs and illegal sales of meat leading to poor sanitary control were all risk factors that were associated with an increased prevalence of cysticercosis in Benin Republic [30] as it will promote sale of infected pork carcass to unsuspecting consumers (since condemnation cannot be carried out) and predispose them to infection by these parasites (taeniasis) which increases transmission of infection in the community while increase age, stigma and lack of medical facilities were associated with increase prevalence of epilepsy, people with epilepsy may hide their true identity due to fear of marginalization and may not get proper health care [31]. In Burkina Faso, being a male, pig farming including percentage of soil in sand, residing in poor homes, lack of latrine. Males may have poor hygiene compared with females as they are likely to eat improperly washed fruits or vegetables after purchase and may eat food from food vendors prepared outside the home who might be carriers of the adult tapeworm. The authors also thought the acidic nature of the gastrointestinal tract might have made the eggs tolerate slightly more acidic soil. The higher soil (sandy) percentage might have favored spread of taenid eggs unto vegetation and water by wind. Carabin et al. [32] and living in communities with higher percentage of traditional pig husbandry [32, 36] were risk factors associated with the seroprevalence of cysticercosis [32]. Other factors include pig ownership, preparation method of pork by mothers, access to latrine [33] and pork consumption, pork consumption is associated with cysticercosis either by self-infection or through ingestion of contaminated food and water [32, 37]. Interestingly, previous consumption of pork, being a paid worker or trader as against farmer and housewives was also associated with the seroprevalence of cysticercosis [22, 37]. It was also observed that free roaming pigs in the rainy season and knowledge of porcine cysticercosis was associated with an increase prevalence of porcine cysticercosis. Free roaming pigs get exposed to infected human feces deposited in the bush or open field thereby increasing the chance of infection and spread of porcine cysticercosis. Being a residence with more than one individual having epilepsy was associated with higher prevalence of active cysticercosis. Refs. [34, 36] observed that NCC and epilepsy were observed in older people compared with people with epilepsy without NCC. In addition, NCC was associated with epilepsy in communities where pig husbandry is practised and higher prevalence of NCC was observed in people with epilepsy. In Ghana, pork consumption and consumption of measly pork and pork soups lightly cooked were risk factors for taeniasis [39], while hypertension and exposure to *Taenia solium* infection were risk factors responsible for adult onset of epilepsy [40]. In Nigeria, pork preparation method and history of epilepsy was associated with seroprevalence of cysticercosis. Heat generated from boiling or frying is likely to kill the metacestode compared with heat from roasting or barbecuing [48]. Others include type and availability of toilets, open defecation, lack of personal hygiene after toilet use, pork consumption and traditional system of pig management [47]. One of the risk factors for epilepsy was history of febrile convulsions [70], purchasing home slaughtered pigs, lack of toilet facilities [64], sourcing pig from the northern part of the country and local breed of pigs [26]. It was observed in Senegal that the risk factor for seropositivity to cysticercosis was older age group and lack of latrine [42].

4. Discussion

Majority of studies on epilepsy use various combination of screening questionnaires, clinical confirmation by neurologists, general practitioners or medical students to identify cases of epilepsy with screening questionnaires developed by World Health Organization (WHO) [72] and Limoges Institute of Epidemiology and Tropical Neurology IENT questionnaire [69]. Epileptic seizures, which are the most common presentation of neurocysticercosis, have been documented in developing countries, which is three to six times higher than those in developed countries [68]. Causes of epilepsy are highly variable across different regions of sub-Saharan Africa and depend on geographical, climatic, political, social and hygienic conditions [73]. The main and most important causes of epilepsy seem to be very similar throughout sub-Saharan Africa showing that hypertension [40]. A genetic predisposition, a past history of febrile convulsions, perinatal neurological disorders, head injuries, cerebrovascular accidents and infections of the central nervous system account for most cases of epilepsy [73] Other presumed causes include witch craft/spiritual [43, 74], brain tumor [75], blood transmission and birth trauma due to self-delivery. Also included are protozoon and helminthic infections, including admission to hospital with malaria, exposure to *T. canis*, *T. gondii*, *O. volvulus* and *T. solium* [40] of which *Taenia solium* has received attention in sub-Saharan Africa over the past few years. Neurocysticercosis is a common cause of epilepsy in pig breeding area [76], however the wide variation in the frequency of epilepsy in the continent could be due to different definitions and type of epilepsy including the population studied and type of sample [44]. Some studies in the region showed the association between epilepsy and cysticercosis using different diagnostic criteria both for epilepsy and cysticercosis. These include three studies in Burkina Faso, of which some researchers [34] showed a seropositivity between cysticercal antigens and active epilepsy with a prevalence odds ratio (POR) of 2.40 (95%). A second study [36] showed 68 of the subjects confirmed with epilepsy by CT scan and 20 were diagnosed with definitive NCC (for a proportion of 45.5–46.9% in two of the study villages). The third study [37] showed that 39 of 70 positive were confirmed with epilepsy for a lifetime prevalence of 4.5% and epilepsy was associated with cysticercosis by Ag-ELISA (POR = 3.1, 95% BCI = 1.0; 8.3). All three studies confirmed epilepsy by ILAE definition/physician. In Senegal, a study [42] showed that one of 10 CT-scan positives individual by Ag-ELISA and EITB was reported to have epileptic seizures, and cerebral CT-scans showed that 23.3% of the seropositive were affected by neurocysticercosis. In Togo, a previous study [57] showed that cysticercosis (confirmed by ELISA, anatomopathological examination, cranial or muscle X-ray) caused 29.5% epilepsy in sufferers. A study by [40] in five Health and Demographic Surveillance System centeres in Kintampo Ghana and four other countries (Kenya, South Africa, Uganda and Tanzania) showed that epilepsy was significantly associated with exposure to *T. solium* (odds ratios 7·03, P = 0·002), in adults epilepsy confirmed by questionnaire/clinician and cysticercosis was confirmed by detection antibody by Western Blot, while active convulsive epilepsy in the study was defined as two or more unprovoked convulsive seizures (occurring at least 24 h apart, with at least one seizure in the preceding 12 months).

The stigmatization and marginalization of epilepsy is also enormous *n* many African countries, epileptic patients are cast out because it is considered a contagious or shameful disease [28, 43, 69, 77]. Those affected go through social seclusion and people will not marry PWE unless both parties have epilepsy. For example, consanguineous marriage is forbidden by culture in South East Nigeria [43], and may potentially force them to intermarry thereby promoting genetic transmission of epilepsy [43, 44]. Other beliefs include that inheriting properties from PWE will get one infected but if a medicine man performs burial rites for the dead person and takes away their properties and burn it then it stops. Burial of PWE far away from home prevents people from getting epilepsy. Eating, sleeping together or wearing same clothes with PWE is said to be a source of infection [43, 44]. Eating of pork by someone with epilepsy promotes cysticercosis and corroborates with a study that found a significant link between cysticercosis occurrence and epilepsy [78]. In West Africa, *T. solium* cysticercosis in pigs and man has been reported and reports have shown the prevalence's of porcine cysticercosis across the west African countries varies from 0.05 to 46% for both carcass inspection and serological studies and prevalence of taeniid eggs were found to be between 8.6 and 40% based on stool microscopy while copro-antigen ELISA gave a prevalence of 30% [65] as shown in **Tables 1** and **2**. Difference in severity of infection caused by *T. solium* could also explain the differences in prevalence of epilepsy. In addition, the extent of the presence of other environmental factors such as use of bad hygiene practices, close contact of humans and pigs and consumption of inadequately cooked pork affects the differences in prevalence of epilepsy [31] including free roaming pigs [43]. Abattoirs and approved slabs are the only approved places for slaughter and inspection of pork meat for consumption, however most carcasses are sold uninspected hence, lack of inspection and large scale clandestine slaughter of pigs promote spread of cysticercosis [32, 34]. The poor knowledge of *T. solium*, poor hand washing practices, not treating drinking water and handling of raw pork with bare hands promote spread of cysticercosis [65]. Reports in the region indicate that home slaughter conditions were normally substandard because they are makeshift and not constructed to actually meet the requirements of ideal slaughter premises [48]. There was also strong association between knowledge of cysticercosis and occupation and could be attributed to the fact that people in certain occupations are considered to be more knowledgeable about the disease than others [48].

5. Conclusions

The high prevalence of porcine and human cysticercosis and epilepsy in the region indicates that there is a need to get more updated prevalence data of cysticercosis in rural areas where epilepsy is suspected to be more prevalent, compared to urban regions due to parasitic infection. Studies determining the association between epilepsy and cysticercosis should be carried out in countries where it has not been done. The conditions necessary for the parasite to thrive and be transmitted in the region is present in West Africa. Interventions studies including Health education has only been done recently in Burkina Faso, such intervention measures should be carried out in other parts of the region so as to enlighten the populace on the menace caused by the parasite and how it could be prevented.

6. Limitations

The present study has some limitations as the criteria for inclusion and exclusion of articles might have increased or reduced the number of studies used in the region and not all risk factor s and causes of epilepsy were discussed. The study did not determine the prevalence of epilepsy and both porcine and human cysticercosis, in the region as the aim of the study was to show data on studies done by other researchers in the region.

Acknowledgements

The authorship criteria are listed in our Authorship Policy: https://www.intechopen.com/page/authorship-policy.

This section of your manuscript may also include funding information.

Conflict of interest

The authors declare no conflict of interest.

Notes/thanks/other declarations

We wish to thank the management of National Veterinary Research Institute Vom for assistance rendered during the preparation of the manuscript.

Acronyms and abbreviations

PWE	people with epilepsy
HCC	human cysticercosis
Ag-ELISA	antigen ELISA
Ab-ELISA	antibody ELISA
ND	not done
GP	general population
VL	villagers
CR	cross sectional survey
CT	computed tomography
HB	hospital based

T. canis	*Toxoca canis*
T. gondii	*Toxoplasma gondii*
O. volvulus	*Onchocerca volvulus*
PC	porcine cysticercosis
TE	taeniasis
BCI	Bayesian hierarchical logistic regression credible intervals

Author details

Rebecca Weka[1*], Pam Luka[1], Ndudim Ogo[1] and Paul Weka[2]

1 National Veterinary Research Institute, Vom, Plateau, Nigeria

2 Ministry of Agriculture and Rural Development, Plateau, Nigeria

*Address all correspondence to: bekkyweka@gmail.com

References

[1] WHO. A Rationale for Investment and Action World Health Organization 2016, WHO/HTM/NTD/NZD/2016; 2016

[2] Gabriël S, Dorny P, Mwape KE, Trevisan C, Braae UC, Magnussen P, et al. Control of *Taenia solium* taeniasis/cysticercosis: The best way forward for sub-Saharan Africa? Acta Tropica. 2016;**165**:252-260

[3] Torgerson PR, Macpherson CN. The socioeconomic burden of parasitic zoonoses: Global trends. Veterinary Parasitology. 2011;**182**:79-95

[4] Fleury A, Sciutto E, de Aluja AS, Carpio A. Cysticercosis: A preventable, but embarrassing neglected disease still prevalent in non-developed countries. In: Zoonoses-Infections Affecting Humans and Animals. Dordrecht: Springer; 2015. pp. 335-354

[5] Lightowlers MW, Assana E, Jayashi CM, Gauci CG, Donadeu M. Sensitivity of partial carcass dissection for assessment of porcine cysticercosis at necropsy. International Journal for Parasitology. 2015;**45**:815-818

[6] Del Brutto OH, García HH. Neurocysticercosis in non endemic countries: Time for a reappraisal. Neuroepidemiology. 2012;**39**:145-146

[7] Lightowlers MW, Garcia HH, Gauci CG, Donadeu M, Abela-Ridder B. Monitoring the outcomes of interventions against *Taenia solium*: Options and suggestions. Parasite Immunology. 2016;**38**:158-169

[8] Trevisan C, Devleesschauwer B, Schmidt V, Winkler AS, Harrison W, Johansen MV. The societal cost of *Taenia solium* cysticercosis in Tanzania. Acta Tropica. 2017a;**165**:141-154

[9] Johansen MV, Trevisan C, Gabriël S, Magnussen P, Braae UC. Are we ready for *Taenia solium* cysticercosis elimination in sub-Saharan Africa? Parasitology. 2016;**144**:59-64

[10] Praet N, Kanobana KC, Maketa V, Lukanu P, Pascal L, Katja P, et al. *Taenia solium* cysticercosis in the Democratic Republic of Congo: How does pork trade affect the transmission of the parasite? PLoS Neglected Tropical Diseases. 2010;**4**(9):e817. DOI: 10.1371/journal.pntd.0000817

[11] Carabin H, Ndimubanzi PC, Budke CM, Nguyen H, Qian Y, Cowan LD, et al. Clinical manifesta-tions associated with neurocysticercosis: A systematic review. PLoS Neglected Tropical Diseases. 2011;**5**:e1152

[12] Carpio A, Hauser WA. Epilepsy in the developing world. Current Neurology and Neuroscience Reports. 2009;**9**:319-326

[13] Prasad KN, Prasad A, Gupta RK, Nath K, Pradhan S, Tripathi M, et al. Neurocysticercosis in patients with active epilepsy from a pig farming community of Lucknov district, North India. Transactions of the Royal Society of Tropical Medicine and Hygiene. 2009;**103**(2):144-150

[14] Preux PM, Druet-Cabanac M. Epidemiology and aetiology of epilepsy in sub-Saharan Africa. Lancet Neurology. 2005;**4**:21-31

[15] Ngugi AK, Bottomley C, Kleinschmidt I, Sander JW, Newton CR. Estimation of the burden of active and life-time epilepsy: A meta-analytic approach. Epilepsia. 2010;**51**:883-890

[16] Ndimubanzi PC, Carabin H, Budke CM, Nguyen H, Qian YJ, Rainwater E, et al. A systematic review of the frequency of neurocyticercosis with a focus on people with epilepsy.

PLoS Neglected Tropical Diseases. 2010;**4**:e870

[17] Carabin H, Krecek RC, Cowan LD, Michael L, Foyaca-Sibat H, Nash T, et al. Estimation of the cost of *Taenia solium* cysticercosis in eastern Cape Province, South Africa. Tropical Medicine and International Health. 2006;**11**:906-916

[18] Weka RP, Kamani J, Cogan T, Eisler M, Morgan ER. Overview of *Taenia solium* cysticercosis in West Africa. Acta Tropica. 2018;**190**:329-338

[19] Geerts S, Nguekam J, Brandt J, Dorny P, Antwerpen N, Science A. The taeniasis-cysticercosis complex in west and Central Africa. Southeast Asian Journal of Tropical Medicine and Public Health. 2004;**35**:262-265

[20] Goussanou SE, Kpodekon TM, Saegerman C, Azagoun E, Youssao AI, Farougou S, et al. Spatial distribution and risks factors of porcine cysticercosis in southern Benin based meat inspection records. International Research Journal of Microbiology. 2013;**4**(8):188-196

[21] Dahourou LD, Ndayikeza C, Savadogo M, Gbati OB. Prevalence and economic losses resulting from parasitic zoonosis on swine and ruminants in Ouagadougou abattoir (Burkina Faso). International Journal of Biological and Chemical Sciences. 2018;**12**(5):2226-2235

[22] Ganaba R, Praet N, Carabin H, Millogo A, Tarnagda Z, Dorny P, et al. Factors associated with the prevalence of circulating antigens to porcine cysticercosis in three villages of Burkina Faso. PLoS Neglected Tropical Diseases. 2011;**5**(1):e927

[23] Gweba M, Faleke OO, Junaidu AU, Fabiyi JP, Fajinmi AO. Some risk factors for *Taenia solium* cysticercosis in semi-intensively raised pigs in Zuru, Nigeria. Veterinaria Italiana. 2010;**46**(1):57-67

[24] Karshima N, Bobbo A, Udokainyang A, Salihu A. *Taenia solium* cysticercosis in pigs slaughtered in IBI local government area of Taraba state, Nigeria. Journal of Animal Science Advances. 2013;**3**(3):103-109

[25] Onah DN, Chiejina SN. *Taenia solium* cysticercosis and human taeniasis in the Nsukka area of Enugu state, Nigeria. Annals of Tropical Medicine and Parasitology. 1995;**89**(4):399-407

[26] Idika I, Njoga A, Eze I, Iheagwam C, Ezenduka E, Njoga E, et al. Re-evaluation of porcine cysticercosis in Nsukka area of Enugu state, Nigeria. Asian Pacific Journal of Tropical Disease. 2017;**7**(9):519-522

[27] Debrock C, Preux P-M, Houinato D, Druet-Cabanac M, Kassa F, Adjien C, et al. Estimation of the prevalence of epilepsy in the Benin region of Zinvié using the capture-recapture method. International Journal of Epidemiology. 2000;**29**(2):330-335

[28] Houinato D, Yemadje LP, Glitho G, Adjien C, Avode G, Druet-Cabanac M, et al. Epidemiology of epilepsy in rural B enin: Prevalence, incidence, mortality, and follow-up. Epilepsia. 2013;**54**(4):757-763

[29] Avode DG, Bouteille B, Houngbe F, Adjien C. Epilepsy, cysticercosis and and neurocysticercosis in Benin. European Neurology. 1998;**39**(1):60

[30] Houinato D, Ramanankandrasana B, Adjidé C, Melakul Z, Josse R, Avodé G, et al. Seroprevalence of cysticercosis in Benin. Transactions of the Royal Society of Tropical Medicine and Hygiene. 1998;**92**:621-624

[31] Yemadje LP, Houinato D, Quet F, Druet-Cabanac M, Preux PM. Understanding the differences in prevalence of epilepsy in tropical regions. Epilepsia. 2011;**52**(8):1376-1381

[32] Carabin H, Millogo A, Cissé A, Gabriël S, Sahlu I, Dorny P, et al. Prevalence of and factors associated with human cysticercosis in 60 villages in three provinces of Burkina Faso. PLoS Neglected Tropical Diseases. 2015;**9**(11):e0004248

[33] Carabin H, Millogo A, Ngowi HA, Bauer C, Dermauw V, Koné AC, et al. Effectiveness of a community-based educational programme in reducing the cumulative incidence and prevalence of human *Taenia solium* cysticercosis in Burkina Faso in 2011-14 (EFECAB): A cluster-randomised controlled trial. The Lancet Global Health. 2018;**6**(4):e411-e425

[34] Sahlu I, Bauer C, Ganaba R, Preux PM, Cowan LD, Dorny P, et al. The impact of imperfect screening tools on measuring the prevalence of epilepsy and headaches in Burkina Faso. PLoS Neglected Tropical Diseases. 2019;**13**(1):e0007109

[35] Sahlu I, Carabin H, Ganaba R, Preux PM, Cissé AK, Tarnagda Z, et al. Estimating the association between being seropositive for cysticercosis and the prevalence of epilepsy and severe chronic headaches in 60 villages of rural Burkina Faso. PLoS Neglected Tropical Diseases. 2018;**13**(1):e0007101

[36] Millogo A, Nitiéma P, Carabin H, Boncoeur-Martel MP, Rajshekhar V, Tarnagda Z, et al. Prevalence of neurocysticercosis among people with epilepsy in rural areas of Burkina Faso. Epilepsia. 2012;**53**(12):2194-2202

[37] Nitiéma P, Carabin H, Hounton S, Praet N, Cowan LD, Ganaba R, et al. Prevalence case-control study of epilepsy in three Burkina Faso villages. Acta Neurologica Scandinavica. 2012;**126**(4):270-278

[38] Debouverie M. Epidemiologie des Syndromes Cpileptiques: A Pro-pos d'une Ctude africaine. Nancy, France: Thkse MCdecine; 1991

[39] Bimi L, Laar AK, Anto F. Prevalence and risk factors of taeniasis in the Bunkpurugu-Yunyoo District of northern Ghana. Journal of Bacteriology and Parasitology. 2012;**3**:129

[40] Ngugi AK, Bottomley C, Kleinschmidt I, Wagner RG, Kakooza-Mwesige A, Ae-Ngibise K, et al. Prevalence of active convulsive epilepsy in sub-Saharan Africa and associated risk factors: Cross-sectional and case-control studies. The Lancet Neurology. 2013;**12**(3):253-263

[41] Goudsmit J, van der Waals FW, Gajdusek C. Epilepsy in the Gbawein and Wroughbarh clan of Grand Bassa county, Liberia: The endemic occurrence of'See-ee'in the native population. Neuroepidemiology. 1983;**2**(1-2):24-34

[42] Secka A, Grimm F, Marcotty T, Geysen D, Niang AM, Ngale V, et al. Old focus of cysticercosis in a senegalese village revisited after half a century. Acta Tropica. 2011;**119**(2-3):199-202

[43] Osakwe C, Otte WM, Alo C. Epilepsy prevalence, potential causes and social beliefs in Ebonyi state and Benue state, Nigeria. Epilepsy Research. 2014;**108**(2):316-326

[44] Ezeala-Adikaibe BA, Orjioke C, Ekenze O, Ijoma U, Onodugo O, Molokwu O, et al. Prevalence of active convulsive epilepsy in an urban slum in Enugu south East Nigeria. Seizure. 2016;**35**:100-105

[45] Babalola O, Adu A, Akano AO. Ocular cysticercosis in a 32-year-old man in Abuja: Ultrasonic features as an aid in diagnosis. Clinical Ophthalmology. 2275;**2013**:7

[46] Mogaji HO, Adeniran AA, Fagbenro MT, Olabinke DB, Abe EM,

Ekpo UF. Prevalence of human taeniasis in Odeda area of Ogun state, Nigeria. International Journal of Tropical Disease and Health. 2016;**17**:1-8

[47] Weka RP, Ikeh EI, Kamani J. Seroprevalence of antibodies (IgG) to *Taenia solium* among pig rearers and associated risk factors in Jos metropolis, Nigeria. Journal of Infection in Developing Countries. 2013;**7**(02):067-072

[48] Edia-Asuke AU, Inabo HI, Mukaratirwa S, Umoh VJ, Whong CM, Asuke S, et al. Seroprevalence of human cysticercosis and its associated risk factors among humans in areas of Kaduna metropolis, Nigeria. Journal of Infection in Developing Countries. 2015;**9**(08):799-805

[49] Omonisi AE, Odujoko OO, Aluko JA, Akinyemi HA, Alatishe OI, Omoniyi-Esan GO. Human cysticercosis of the breast mimicking breast cancer: A report of a case from Ile-Ife, Nigeria. Nigerian Journal of Medicine: Journal of the National Association of Resident Doctors of Nigeria. 2014;**23**(4):351-354

[50] Uhumwangho OM, Ugiagbe EE. Cysticercosis in the anterior chamber: A case report. West African Journal of Medicine. 2012;**31**(4):270-272

[51] Osuntokun BO, Adeuja AO, Nottidge VA, Bademosi O, Olumide A, Ige O, et al. Prevalence of the epilepsies in Nigerian Africans: A community-based study. Epilepsia. 1987;**28**(3):272-279

[52] Ndoye NF, Sow AD, Diop AG, Sessouma B, Sene-Diouf F, Boissy L, et al. Prevalence of epilepsy its treatment gap and knowledge, attitude and practice of its population in sub-urban Senegal an ILAE/IBE/WHO study. Seizure. 2005;**14**(2):106-111

[53] N'Diaye Epid Cmiologie des Cpilepsies au SCnCgal. 7th Meeting of the Pan-African Assoc. of Neural. Abidjan: Science; 1986

[54] Gerrits C. A west African epilepsy focus. Lancet. 1983;**1**:358

[55] Diagana M, Preux PM, Tuillas M, Ould Hamady A, Druet-Cabanac M. Dépistage de l'épilepsie en zones tropicales: validation d'un questionnaire en Mauritanie. Bulletin de la Société de Pathologie Exotique. 2006;**99**(2):103-107

[56] Balogou AA, Grunitzky KE, Beketi KA, Bouteille B, Dumas M. Cysticercosis and epilepsy in the city of tone, north of Togo. Revue Neurologique. 2000;**156**(3):270-273

[57] Dumas M. Cysticercose et neurocysticercose: enquête épidémiologique dans le nord du Togo. Bulletin de la Société de Pathologie Exotique. 1990;**83**:263-274

[58] Coulibaly ND, Yameogo KR. Prevalence and control of zoonotic diseases: Collaboration between public health workers and veterinarians in Burkina Faso. Acta Tropica. 2000;**76**(1):53-57

[59] Atawalna J, Ewura S, Mensah M. Prevalence and financial losses associated with porcine cysticercosis in the Kumasi metropolis of Ghana. International Journal of Livestock Research. 2015;**5**(9):21-26

[60] Permin A, Yelifari L, Bloch P, Steenhard N, Hansen NP, Nansen P. Parasites in cross-bred pigs in the upper east region of Ghana. Veterinary Parasitology. 1999;**87**(1):63-71

[61] Cadmus SI, Adesokan HK, Awosanya AE. Public health issues and observations made during meat inspection at Bodija municipal abattoir, Ibadan, Oyo state, Nigeria. Nigerian Veterinary Journal. 2008; **29**(2):43-47

[62] Biu AA, Ijudai J. Prevalence and morphometric studies on porcine cysticercosis in Adamawa state, Nigeria. Sokoto Journal of Veterinary Sciences. 2012;**10**(1):28-31

[63] Agere H, Bemgba E, Iorgema U. Prevalence of Cysticercosis in Pigs Slaughtered in Jalingo, Nigeria. 2016;**1**(2):578-581

[64] Adesokan HK, Adeoye FA. Porcine cysticercosis in slaughtered pigs and factors related to *Taenia solium* transmission amongst abattoir workers in Ibadan, Nigeria. The Pan African Medical Journal. 2019;**32**:145

[65] Edia-Asuke AU, Inabo HI, Umoh VJ, Whong CM, Asuke S, Edeh RE. Assessment of sanitary conditions of unregistered pig slaughter slabs and post mortem examination of pigs for *Taenia solium* metacestodes in Kaduna metropolis, Nigeria. Infectious Diseases of Poverty. 2014;**3**(1):45

[66] Weka RP, Ikeh EI. Seroprevalence of cysticercosis and intestinal parasitism in pigs in Jos Metropolis. Journal of Animal and Veterinary Advances. 2009;**8**:883-887

[67] Secka A, Marcotty T, De Deken R, Van Marck E, Geerts S. Porcine cysticercosis and risk factors in the Gambia and Senegal. Journal of Parasitology Research. 2010

[68] Commissionon Epidemiology and Prognosis, International League Against Epilepsy. Guidelines for epidemiologic studies on epilepsy. Epilepsia. 1993;**34**:592-596

[69] Preux PM, Druet-Cabanac M, Debrock C, Tapie PH, Dumas M, et al. Comitde Recherchesurl' Epilepsiedel' Institutd' Epidmiologie Neurologiqueetde Neurologie Tropicalede Limoges. Bulletin de la Société de Pathologie Exotique. 2000;**93**:276-278

[70] Nwani PO, Nwosu MC, Asomugha LA, Enwereji KO, Arinzechi EO, Ogunniyi AO. Epidemiology of active epilepsy in a suburban community in Southeast Nigeria: A door-to-door survey. Nigerian Journal of Clinical Practice. 2015;**18**(4):527-533

[71] Adegbehingbe BO, Soetan EO, Adeoye AO. Case report: intraocular cysticercosis. West African Journal of Medicine. 2003;**22**(4):354-355

[72] Placencia M, Sander JW, Shorvon SD, Ellison RH, Cascante SM. Validation of a screening questionnaire for the detection of epileptic seizuresinepidemiologicalstudies. Brain. 1992;**115**:783-794

[73] Winkler AS. Epilepsy and neurocysticercosis in sub-Saharan Africa. In: Foyaca Sibat H, editor. Novel Aspects on Cysticercosis and Neurocysticercosis. Vol. 30. Rijeka, Croatia: IntechOpen; 2013. pp. 307-340

[74] Eseigbe EE, Sheikh TL, Nuhu FT. Childhood epilepsy in a tropical child psychiatric unit: Challenges of providing care in a resource-constrained environment. Annals of African Medicine. 2013;**12**(4):236

[75] Ogunrin OA, Adeyekun A, Adudu P. Etiologies of epilepsy and health-seeking itinerary of patients with epilepsy in a resource poor setting: Analysis of 342 Nigerian Africans. Seizure. 2013;**22**(7):572-576

[76] Phiri IK, Ngowi H, Afonso S, Matenga E, Boa M, Mukaratirwa S, et al. The emergence of *Taenia solium* cysticercosis in eastern and southern Africa as a serious agricultural problem and public health risk. Acta Tropica. 2003;**87**(1):13-23

[77] Adewuya AO. Parental psychopathology and self-rated quality

of life in adolescents with epilepsy in Nigeria. Developmental Medicine and Child Neurology. 2006;**48**:600-603

[78] Quet F, Rafael F, Ngoungou EB, Diagana M, Druet-Cabanac M, Preux PM. Investigating epilepsy in Africa: 10 years of data collection using a standardized questionnaire in 2,269 peoples with epilepsy. Epilepsia. 2011;**52**(10):1868-1876

Chapter 4

Echinococcus granulosus

Khadeeja Abees Hmood Al-Khalidi, Hiba Riyadh Al-Abodi, Hayder Kamil Jabbar and Baheeja A. Hmood

Abstract

Echinococcus granulosus is also called the hydatid worm, which a parasite that infects humans and animals. It causes zoonotic disease known as echinococcosis (hydatidosis). Adult worms live in the intestines of dogs that are the definitive host. Hydatidosis is known since ancient times and is one of the epidemic diseases that is dangerous to humans in terms of health and economy in most countries of the world. Hydatidosis or echinococcosis unilocular is common in many Arab countries, including Libya, Sudan, Egypt, Lebanon, Syria, Algeria, Palestine, Iraq, and others as well as North, East, and South Africa, Western and Southern Europe, and South America. Studies indicate that the disease is spreading in areas that were previously completely free of it such as North America and Canada. It was also noted that the incidence of the disease in rural areas is close to 50%, and this is due to the large breeding of farm animals and the presence of meat eaters, which helps to complete the life cycle of this parasite, which needs the intermediate host (farm animals and humans) and the definitive host (Canidae).

Keywords: *E. granulosus*, hydatid worm, echinococcosis, hydatidosis, zoonotic disease

1. Introduction

Echinococcus granulosus is one of cestodes that caused cystic hydatid disease (Echinococcosis), and this parasite is transmitted from carnivores (dogs, foxes, leopards, lions, and hyenas), which are the definitive hosts of *E. granulosus* and the parasite (the adult stages) lives in their intestines, to herbivores (sheep, goats, camels, cows, buffaloes, horses, donkeys, pigs, rabbits, and humans), which are intermediate hosts of the parasite where the larvae (hydatid cyst) live [1].

E. granulosus has three different stages of development: eggs, larvae, and adult worms, which are small and do not exceed 7 mm in length as shown in **Figure 1** and live adjacent to the mucous layer of the small intestine of the definitive hosts until they reach the adult phases of sexual maturity in about 5–4 weeks [2, 3]. The adult worm has a spherical head of 0.3 mm diameter with a short neck and three types of connected segments, and the head contains a sucker surrounded by two rows of spines ranging from 50 to 28 forks, with four side suckers. The segment that follows the head is immature and contains immature genitals, while the middle segment is mature and contains the testes and ovaries and is located in the middle of the genital opening [4, 5]. The third segment is called gravid segment and contains a branched uterus and has 15–12 branches containing 1000–500 eggs [6].

 IntechOpen

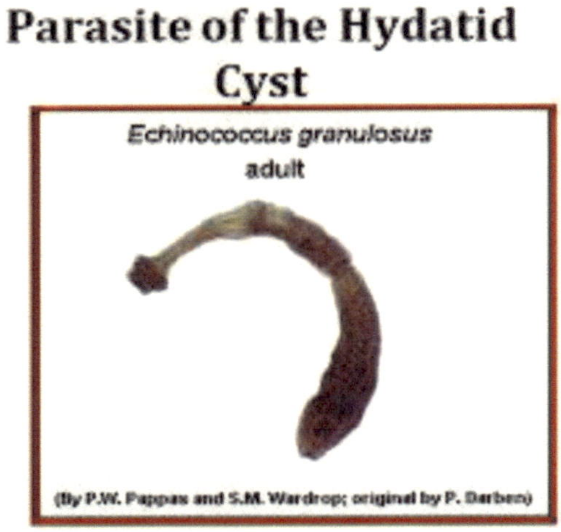

Figure 1.
E. granulosus *adult.*

2. *E. granulosus* eggs

The eggs are spherical in shape (**Figure 2**) and have a diameter of about 40–30 μm and are similar in appearance to the eggs of other tapeworms, containing a hexacanth or oncosphere embryo because the embryo has sixth-hooks lets. The eggs are surrounded by clear coatings [8] and the eggs contain a sticky layer that adheres to the fur of animals and other things, which helps them to spread, as well as insects such as flies, beetles, and birds that play the role of mechanical carrier of eggs, in case of optimal conditions, the eggs remain viable for weeks or months in pastures and gardens as well as they remain viable with the right humidity and moderate temperatures, and the eggs are found in water and wet sand for 3 weeks at 30°C and 225 days at 6°C and 32 days at 10–21°C, also the eggs remain for a short time when exposed to sunlight and dry conditions and kill eggs when exposed to 3.75% of sodium hypochlorite for 10 minutes as well as killed when frozen at −70°C for 4 days or −80°C for 2 days or by heat larger from 60°C for 3 minutes [9].

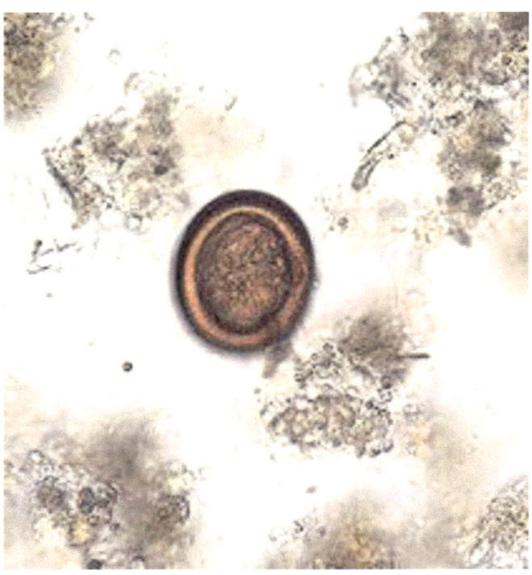

Figure 2.
E. granulosus *egg in feces [7].*

3. Larval stage (hydatid cyst)

When intermediate hosts (farm animals) or humans (accidental host) ingest the eggs, the embryo (oncospheres) hatches and becomes active, transmitted by the bloodstream to the liver or any other organ. As soon as the hexacanth embryo reaches its definitive position, it develops into unilocular hydatid cyst that enlarges and produces daughter cysts or protoscoleces inside the inner layer of the hydatid cyst [10, 11].

4. Transmission

Transmission to humans is caused by fecal-oral route while eating food and water contaminated with parasite eggs, and these eggs are thrown out with feces of the definitive hosts such as dogs or through contamination of hands with eggs found in contaminated soil or sand or in the hair of infected dogs. The definitive hosts become infected with the adult worm when they feed on the hydatid cysts, which are found in the organs of the intermediate host, such as infected sheep [9, 11].

5. Strains of *E. granulosus*

Species of *E. granulosus* is divided into several strains such as G1–G10 and these strains have a high degree of adaptation to their hosts, as these strains are named according to the names of their intermediate hosts that play an important role in the continuity of the life cycle of these strains. These strains vary in shape, rate of development, pathogenicity, and geographical extent of their presence: G1 is found in sheep, G2 in Tasmania sheep, and G3 in buffalo. These strains all fall within the *E. granulosus* species, and G4 strain in equine is therefore called *E. equinus*; G5 in cows is called *E. ortleppi*; G6 in camels; G7 in pigs; G9, which is characterized weak, has been isolated from cystic disease in human cases in Poland; G7, G8, and G9 may fall into *E. canadensis*, and some researchers consider the G9 strain a type of G7 strain in pigs [12].

6. Parasite classification

The classification of Echinococcus genus has been controversial for a long time, and 16 species and 13 subspecies of this genus have been described, based on the difference in the structural and phenotypic properties of the parasite and the characteristics of the host and its type, but only 4 of them are taxonomically adopted: *E. granulosus*, *E. multilocularis*, *E. oligarthrus*, and *E. vogeli* [13]. According to [14], the classification system of granulocytic parasitic parasite is as follows:

Kingdom: Animalia
Phylum: Platyhelminthes
Superclass: Eucestoda
Class: Cestoda
Subclass: Cestoda
Order: Cyclophyllidea (Ben; Braun, 1900)
Family: Taeniidae (Ludwig, 1886)

Genus: Echinococcus (Rud, 1801)
Species: granulosus (Batsch, 1786)

7. The life cycle of the parasite

The adult phases of the *E. granulosus* lives in the mucous layer of the definitive host's small intestine, and the eggs are highly resistant to harsh environmental conditions for several months or even a year depending on environmental conditions [15]. Therefore, it remains a source of infection to the intermediate hosts during drinking contaminated water and food, including humans that may also be infected by contact with infected dogs, especially in children, whereas eggs adhere to dog hair around the anus [16, 17].

The eggs reach the stomach of the intermediate host and then decompose the chitinous cortex by digestive juices and release the embryo (oncospheres) of the sixth-hooks, and the oncospheres penetrate the intestine and reach the liver, lungs, and other organs including the brain and muscles to develop into hydatid cysts at the end of about 5 months [18].

When the definitive host feeds on infected organs of the intermediate host, the parasite will reach its small intestine, where the primary heads grow into adult worms within 7–4 weeks, and each worm produces thousands of eggs per day, starting the cycle again [15] (**Figure 3**).

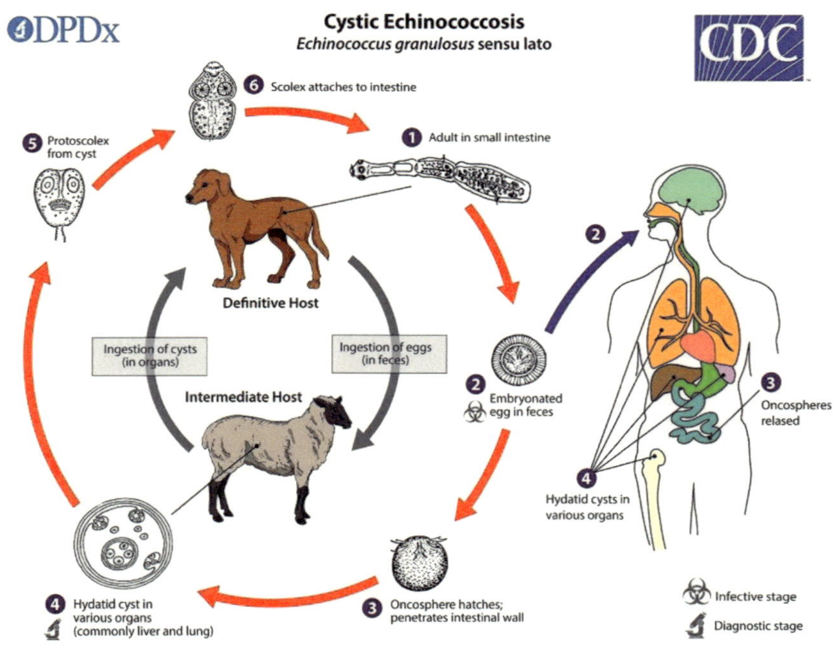

Figure 3.
The adult E. granulosus *(sensu lato) (2–7 mm long)* ❶ *resides in the small intestine of the definitive host. Gravid proglottids release eggs* ❷ *that are passed in the feces and are immediately infectious. After ingestion by a suitable intermediate host, eggs hatch in the small intestine and release six-hooked oncospheres* ❸ *that penetrate the intestinal wall and migrate through the circulatory system into various organs, especially the liver and lungs. In these organs, the oncosphere develops into a thick-walled hydatid cyst* ❹ *that enlarges gradually, producing protoscolices and daughter cysts that fill the cyst interior. The definitive host becomes infected by ingesting the cyst-containing organs of the infected intermediate host. After ingestion, the protoscolices* ❺ *evaginate, attach to the intestinal mucosa*❻*, and develop into adult stages* ❶ *in 32–80 days. Humans are aberrant intermediate hosts and become infected by ingesting eggs* ❷*. Oncospheres are released in the intestine* ❸*, and hydatid cysts develop in a variety of organs* ❹*. If cysts rupture, the liberated protoscolices may create secondary cysts in other sites within the body (secondary echinococcosis) [19].*

8. Structure of hydatid cyst (larval stage)

The hydatid cysts (**Figure 4**) of *E. granulosus* are often spherical or semispherical if not compressed by adjacent organs. The size of the hydatid cysts varies with age, approximately 15–1 cm^3 [21].

8.1 The outer (pericyst) layer

The outer layer is also called adventitia or ectocyst that encases the hydatid cyst, and this layer is produced by the host cells (modified dense fibrous protective tissue) as the host's response to the infection. There is a close interaction between the host tissue and the parasite, and this layer plays an important role in the development and survival of the cyst. Any degradation of the outer layer leads to the degeneration or explosion of the hydatid cyst; the diameters of a pericyst layer vary depending on the host organ where the hydatid is present, but in general, the diameters are about a few millimeters [22].

8.2 Laminated (medial) layer

It is a solid, noncellular chitinous layer, white in color, consisting of microfibers fibers and dense granules rich in amino carbohydrates observed under electron microscopy [23]. It plays a role in protecting the parasite from the immune response of host and providing the suitable environment for its continued growth in addition to its role in reducing the effect of drugs used in the treatment of the disease [6].

8.3 Germinal (inner) layer

This is the inner layer of hydatid cyst, a cellular living layer containing nuclei and associated with the lamellar layer by fingerprints formed by the germinal layer [20, 24]. It acts to protect components of the cyst and controls the osmotic pressure of the cyst wall [25]. The buds are formed from the germinal layer and grow toward the cavity of the cyst, and after the buds become vacuolated and stalked, the process of forming buds from the inner layer of cells begins from

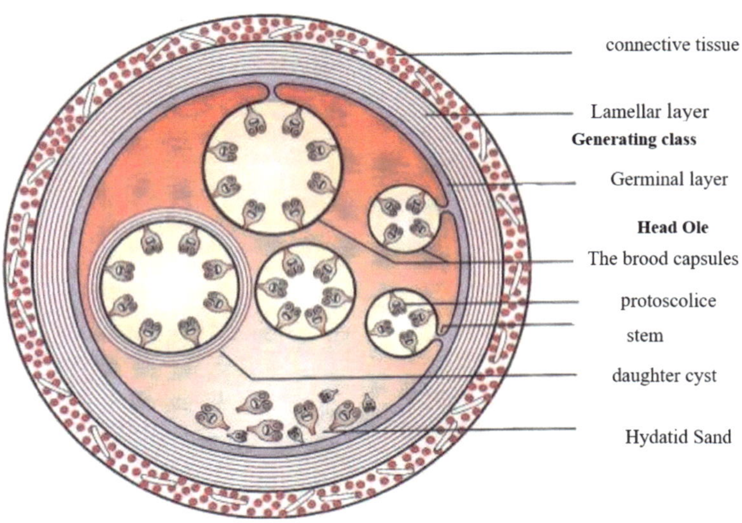

Figure 4.
Cross section in the hydatid cyst [20].

those cavities that lead to the formation of protoscolices [26]. The fertility of the aqueous cyst is determined by the presence of protoscolices, their increasing growth, and their association with the germinal layer, as well as other criteria for determining the cyst fertility through the white color and thickness of the germinal layer [27].

9. Components of hydatid cyst

9.1 Daughter vesicles (brood capsules)

These capsules consist of the generated layer by several endogenous budding, which are small buds formed from the germinal layer toward the cavity of the cyst [15]. These buds enlarge, and each capsule is connected to the germinal layer of the parental cyst by the stem. The process of budding is repeated, and each capsule contains large numbers of protoscolices, which have about 30–10 heads per capsule [28]; capsules are gradually separated from the germinal layer and float in the cyst fluid. These capsules are similar in their structure to the parental cyst [29].

The capsules may rupture and protoscolices may be released together with the free capsules, and this is the so-called hydatid sand. Occasionally, cysts are free from brood capsules when they grow in an inappropriate medium or due to bacterial invasion or calcification. The capsules are formed but do not produce protoscolices, and these are called sterile cysts, whereas capsules that produce protoscolices are called fertile cysts [14].

9.2 Hydatid sand

A term of hydatid sand refers to the contents of the hydatid cyst, which includes the daughter cysts, brood capsules, and protoscolices that present in the hydatid fluid of the *E. granulosus* [30].

9.3 Hydatid cyst fluid

It is a clear colorless or yellowish liquid with a specific weight of 1.005–1.009, a pH of 7.2–6.7, and inorganic substances such as iron, chlorine, magnesium, sodium, calcium, cadmium, nickel, chromium, copper, and some enzymes such as glutamic pyruvic transaminase (GTP), glutamic oxaloacetic transaminase (GOT), Acid phosphatase with lipase, oxidase, phosphatase, and dehydrate enzymes. They vary in quantity and quality depending on the source of the parasite and the location of the cyst and metabolism of parasites such as ammonia, bilirubin, and creatinine [31].

10. Epidemiology of *E. granulosus*

The *E. granulosus* parasite spreads almost all over the world, but it is more common in rural areas with large pastoral areas, where there are large numbers of animals that are hosts of the parasite, such as cattle, sheep, and others, with the presence of definitive hosts in these areas especially dogs [32]. Echinococcosis is a health and economic problem in most parts of the world and some studies have recorded more than 50 cases per 100,000 people annually in high endemic areas, where the prevalence of the disease in China, Argentina, and East Africa was about 5–10%. The disease also kills about 1 million people a year around the world and also causes a loss of about $3 billion, including treatment and livestock expenses [15, 33].

It is also highly endemic in parts of Africa, Europe, Australia, Asia, and the Mediterranean countries [34], as well as Middle Eastern countries including Iran, Saudi Arabia, Kuwait, Jordan, Palestine, Syria, Lebanon, and Iraq [35]. The epidemiology of the disease depends on the economic and agricultural factors and the level of learning and health and social culture in the human society where the parasite is spread, and what helps to spread the disease is the mixing with pets, especially dogs, in the absence of appropriate health conditions [36].

Iraq is a highly endemic country for the disease, due to the spread of loose parasite-infected dogs [37]. Although there are many recent studies of the epidemic of this disease, it is still a major health problem and is still endemic in Iraq, where there were not enough attempts to combat it despite the availability of modern conditions and equipment for diagnosis and treatment [38].

Epidemiology of hydatosis and cystic type (CE) is still on the rise due to its global distribution and high regional prevalence, and alveolar type (AE) has been observed during the past two decades and a decrease in the rate of morbidity and mortality, especially in Asia, as a result of intensive studies of epidemiology in all countries of the world [39].

11. Hydatidosis (Echinococcosis)

Hydatidosis is one of the oldest known diseases of the human being. This disease was described by the Egyptians in a document dating back to 1534 BC, as mentioned by the Babylonians in the Bible Talmud. It described the cyst as a bladder filled with fluid [40]. This disease arises from the formation of hydatid cysts of different sizes in different locations such as the liver and lungs in both animals and humans, and the severity of the disease depends on the number of cysts, size, and location. These cysts may lead to loss of human life in addition to economic losses in the field of livestock; the incidence of this disease is high in humans because its risk is that it is detected only by chance during radiological examinations or various surgical operations, but in animals, it is discovered during routine detection in massacres [1].

The cause of hydatidosis disease is due to two important factors. The first is that it is not possible to know the infection in the early stages since the onset of the disease because it does not show symptoms until the cyst has increased in size of the cyst, which puts pressure on the adjacent tissues [41]. The second factor is the loss of therapeutic means, and the disease is very similar to the severity of its metastasis in the metastasis stage [42]. These cysts are found in all parts of the body except hair and nails [43].

This disease is one of the endemic diseases in Iraq and it has an economic, social and health impact on the human, so conducted many studies and research to investigate methods of treatment, which surgical intervention is the most important of these methods, although the patient is exposed to many problems during surgery which may be difficult to perform at times and cannot be performed at other times [44, 45], or the patient is not surgically qualified or as a result of other serious diseases such as immune compromised patients or because of age or anesthesia or the occurrence of the cyst in places difficult for the surgeon to deal with, such as in the cysts of the heart, brain or spine, so the importance of the use of extracts of a different chemical nature treatment of aquatic cyst disease [46].

12. Clinical symptoms of hydatidosis

Hydatis cyst disease (HCD) is slow at the onset of infection and unseen due to slow growth and development of the cyst, which reaches a diameter of about 10–1 mm per year [33]. The appearance of clinical signs depends on the location of the affected organ, the size of the cyst, its location within the affected organ, the stages of its development, and the fertility of its components with the interaction between the related cysts between adjacent organs, especially between the hepatic vessels and bile ducts [47]. In humans, the symptoms are dependent on the affected organ, and the liver is the most exposed organ, with a rate of about 70–60%, followed by lungs 22–20%, spleen, heart, muscles, eye, and thyroid gland 6%, and the kidneys, brain, and bones 1% and don't hardly any organ of body free from hydatid cyst except teeth, nails and hair [48].

Symptoms in the liver are: an enlarged, and it becomes sensitive when palpated with liver abscesses, in addition abdominal pain, vomiting and nausea, as well as an increase in hepatic blood pressure and in cavity of the lower vena cava also there secondary fibrosis in the ducts bile, the hydatid cyst causes significant pressure on the diaphragm when adhesion to it and leads to a breach and exit of the contents of the cyst in the chest [49]. In the lung, clinical symptoms depend on the size of the cyst and its condition whether it is healthy or torn, causing the presence of pressure of cyst inside the lobes of the lung [50] with varying severity of chest pain and coughing, hemoptysis, shortness of breath, and hemorrhage, and in the lungs, these symptoms do not appear at the first sight of the disease [51–53]. When the cyst penetrates into the pulmonary vesicles, it is a suitable environment for fungal and bacterial infections, leading to pneumonia after infection and thus destroying the lung [54].

The explosion of the hydatid cyst inside the abdominal cavity leads to a shock known as anaphylactic shock due to acute allergic reactions, and this shock leads to the severe spread of secondary cysts in the affected organ and adjacent organs, and is sometimes followed by the explosion of the cyst at any site within the body leaking its contents into the blood circulation that leads to headaches and other complications that may lead to sudden death [28].

The symptoms develop even when the cyst is small, and most cases of cerebral cyst disease were diagnosed in children [11]. This infection is serious that sometimes it leads to death; cysts in the eye are rare and cause an external tumor of the eye, dysfunction of vision, exophthalmoses, and sometimes blindness around the eyelid [17].

In the bones, cystic hydatid disease often leads to fracture because of the gradual erosion of the cortex and shows symptoms in the form of pain in the upper and lower extremities, and bone bags are abnormal in the form where the laminar layer does not form [55].

In animals, the infection is hidden, and they may be slaughtered sometimes before the onset of symptoms [56]. The severity of the symptoms varies depending on the severity of the disease and the location of the hydatid cyst. Clinical signs generally appear in the affected animal such as decrease in milk production, poor wool, and organ damage in the affected area [57, 58].

13. Conclusion

The current review included the identification of the *E. granulosus* worm and its intermediate and final hosts. The canine family represents the final host, while the human and farm animals represent the intermediate hosts. Several strains of *E. granulosus* were also observed such as G1, G2, G3, G4, G5, G6, G7, G8, G9, and G10.

Acknowledgements

The authors thank the Central Library, Library College of Science/University of Al-Qadisiyah, for providing them with the references adopted in this chapter.

Author details

Khadeeja Abees Hmood Al-Khalidi[1*], Hiba Riyadh Al-Abodi[1], Hayder Kamil Jabbar[2] and Baheeja A. Hmood[2]

1 Department of Environment, College of Sciences, University of AL-Qadisiyah, Iraq

2 Department of Medical and Basic Science, College of Nursing, University of AL-Qadisiyah, Iraq

*Address all correspondence to: khadeeja.abees@qu.edu.iq; khadeejaalkhalidi@gmail.com

References

[1] Arafa MI. Hydatids vesicular disease in humans and animals, the growing disease in the spread. Assiut Journal of Environmental Studies. 2003;(12):181-188

[2] Siracusano A, Delunardo F, Teggi A, Ortona E. Cystic echinococcosis: Aspects of immune response, immunopathogenesis and immune evasion from the human host. Endocrine, Metabolic & Immune Disorders—Drug Targets. 2012;**12**(1):16-23

[3] Mandal S, Mandal MD. Human cystic echinococcosis: Epidemiologic, zoonotic, clinical, diagnostic and therapeutic aspects. Asian Pacific Journal of Tropical Medicine. 2012;**5**(4):253-260

[4] Brozova A, Jankovska I, Bejcek V, Nechybova S, Perinkova P, Horakova B, et al. *Echinococcus* spp.: Tapeworms that pose a danger to both animals and humans—A review. Scientia Agriculturae Bohemica. 2017;**48**(8):193-201

[5] Patkowski W, Krasnodebski M, Grat M, Masior L, Krawczyk M. Surgical treatment of hepatic *Echinococcus granulosus*. Przegląd Gastroenterologiczny. 2017;**12**(3):199-202

[6] Al-Qaisi GHJ. The effect of immune activation in reducing the pathogenicity *Echinococcus granulosus* in mice [master thesis]. Faculty of Education, University of Diyala

[7] Available from: https://en.wikipedia.org/wiki/Echinococcosis

[8] John DT, Petri WA. Markell and Voge's Medical Parasitology. 9th ed. United States of America: Elsevier; 2006. 468p

[9] Krauss H, Weber A, Appel M, Enders B, Isenberg H, Schiefer HG, et al. Parasitic zoonoses. In: Zoonoses: Infectious Diseases Transmissible from Animals to Humans. 3rd ed. Washington, DC: ASM Press; 2003. pp. 334-343

[10] Badley AD, Steckelberg JM, Wilson WR. Cestodes. In: Wilson WR, Sande MA, editors. Current Diagnostics and Treatment in Infectious Diseases. United States: McGraw Hill; 2001

[11] Moro P, Schantz PM. Echinococcosis: A review. International Journal of Infectious Diseases. 2009;**13**(2):125-133

[12] Centers for Disease Control and Prevention (CDC). Available from: http://www.dpd.cdc.gov/dpdx/HTML/Echinococcosis.htm, https://www.cdc.gov/dpdx/az.html, https://www.cdc.gov/dpdx/echinococcosis/index.html

[13] McManus DP. Current status of the genetics and molecular taxonomy of *Echinococcus* sp. Parasitology. 2013;**140**(13):1617-1623

[14] Rahman WA, Elmajdoub LE, Noor S, Wajidi MF. Present status on the taxonomy and morphology of *Echinococcus granulosus*. 2015

[15] Higuita NIA, Brunetti E, McCloskey C. Cystic echinococcosis (Review). Journal of Clinical Microbiology. 2016;**54**(3):518-523

[16] Yang S, Zhao Y, McManus DP, Yang Y. Current research advance on Echinococcosis. In: Echinococcosis. IntechOpen; 2017. pp. 9-23

[17] Thatte S, Thatte S. Ocular hydatid cyst. Annals of Clinical Pathology. 2016;**4**(5):1-5

[18] FAO Manual on Meat Inspection for Developing Countries. Available from: http://www.fao.org/docrep/003/t0756e/t0756e00.htm

[19] Available from: https://www.cdc.gov/parasites/echinococcosis/biology.html

[20] Thompson RCA, McManus DP. In: Eckert J, Gemmell MA, Keslin FX, Pawlawski S, editors. Aetiology: Parasite and Live-cycles. 2001

[21] Salhi SFC. Study of biochemical changes in serum of sheep with hydatosis disease in liver [higher diploma]. College of Veterinary Medicine, University of Al-Qadisiyah; 2011

[22] Golzari SEJ, Sokouti M. Pericyst: The outermost layer of hydatid cyst. World Journal of Gastroenterology. 2014;**20**(5):1377-1378

[23] Muller N, Frei E, Nunez S, Gottstein B. Improved serodiagnosis of alveolar echinococcosis of humans using an in vitro-produced *Echinococcus multilocularis* antigen. Parasitology. 2007;**134**(6):879-888

[24] Arora K. Liver and intrahepatic bile ducts—Nontumor infection infectious (nonviral) disorders. Echinococcal cyst. 2017. Retrieved from: http://www.pathologyoutlines.com/liver.html

[25] Al-Omari MM. Effect of stamper and myrtle extracts on the vitality and growth of *Echinococcus granulosus* primates of human and sheep origin and growth in vivo [master thesis]. College of Education, Mosul University; 2005

[26] Mario G, Mjulieta G, Norbel G. *Echinococcus granulosus* protoscolex formation in natural infections. Biological Research. 2002;**35**(3-4)

[27] Bortoletti G, Ferrett G. Ultrastructural aspects of fertile and sterile cysts of *Echinococcus granulosus* developed in hosts of different species. International Journal for Parasitology. 1978;**8**:421-443

[28] Bogitsh BJ, Carter CE, Oeltmann TN. Human Parasitology. Academic Press; 2013. pp. 254-265

[29] Mehlhorn H. Encyclopedic Reference of Parasitology. Berlin: Springer; 2008

[30] Chiou MT, Wang F-I, Chang PH, Liu C-H, Jeng CR, Cheng CH, et al. Hydatidosis in a Chapman's zebra (*Equus burchelli antiquorum*). Journal of Veterinary Diagnostic Investigation. 2001;**13**:534-537

[31] Taher AJ. Blood, biochemical and immunological study of patients with echinococcosis [master thesis]. College of Education (Ibn Al Haytham), University of Baghdad; 2009

[32] Craig PS, Li T, Qiu J, Zhen R, Wang Q, Giraudoux P, et al. Echinococcosis and Tibetan communities. Emerging Infectious Disease. 2008;**14**(10):1674-1675

[33] Pakala T, Molina M, Wu GY. Hepatic echinococcal cysts. Journal of Clinical and Translational Hepatology. 2016;**4**(1):39-48

[34] McManus DP, Gray DJ, Zhang W, Yang Y. Diagnosis, treatment, and management of Echinococcosis. British Medical Journal. 2012;**344**(7861):39-44

[35] Nasrieh MA, Abdel-Hafez SK, Kamhawi SA. Cystic echinococcosis in Jorden: Socioeconomic evaluation and risk factors. Parasitology Research. 2003;**90**:456-466

[36] Al-Shahwani TA. The effect of some plant extracts on the vitality of protoscoleces of *E. granulosus* of sheep origin and its growth within vivo [master thesis]. University of Mosul; 2010. 160 p

[37] Kshash QH. Study of some epidemiological aspect of important endemic parasitic diseases in

Al-Qadisiyah province. Basrah Journal of Veterinary Research. 2005;**4**(2):72-79

[38] Al-Saimary IE, Al-Shemari MN, Al-Fayadh MMA. Epidemiological and immunological findings on human hydatidosis. Journal of Medical Practice and Review. 2010;**1**:26-34

[39] Deplazes P, Rinaldi L, Alvarez Rojas CA, Torgerson PR, Harandi MF, Romig T, et al. Global distribution of alveolar and cystic echinococcosis. Advances in Parasitology. 2017;**95**:315-493

[40] Sabau AD. Laparoscopic Surgery for Hepatic Hydatid Cyst. Lucian Blaga University of Sibiu, Victor Papilian Faculty of Medicine; 2011

[41] Andersen FI, Tolly HD, Shantz PM, Ding Z. Cystic echinococcosis in the Xinjiang/Uygur Autonomous Region, People's Republic of China. II. Comparison of three levels of a local preventive and control program. The Journal of Tropical Medicine and Parasitology. 1991;**42**:1-10

[42] Novak M. Efficacy of mitomycin against alveolar *Echinococcus*. International Journal for Parasitology. 1990;**20**:119-120

[43] Al-Gharawi AKH. Phenotypic study to determine some strains of *Echinococcus granulosus* in sheep, cows and goats in Salah al-Din Governorate, Iraq [master thesis]. College of Education, Tikrit University; 2004. p. 88

[44] Mentes A, Yalaz S, Killi R, Altintas N. Radical treatment for hepatic echinococcosis. HPB. 2000;**2**(1):49-54

[45] Elissondo MC, Dopchiz MC, Denegri G. Human hydatidosis in Mar del Plata, Buenos Aires Province, Argentina (1992-1995): A preliminary study. Parasitología Latinoamericana. 2002;**57**:124-128

[46] Al-Humairi AKO. Evaluation of efficacy of *Datura stramonium* seed extract on growth and development of hydatid cysts of *E. granulosus* protein cysts in Balb/c eggs (Pharmacological, Histological and Immunological Study) [PhD thesis]. Faculty of Science, University of Kufa; 2010. p. 2

[47] Ammann R, Eckert J. Clinical diagnosis and treatment of Echinococcosis in humans. In: Thompson RCA, Lymbery AJ, editors. *Echinococcus* and Hydatid Disease. Wallingford, UK: CAB International; 1995. pp. 411-451

[48] Marquardt WC, Demaree RS, Grieve RB. Parasitology and Vector Biology. 1st ed. London: Harcourt/Academic Press; 2000

[49] Brunetti E. Echinococcosis hydatid cyst medication. Medscape. 2015. Retrieved from: http://emedicine.medscape.com/article/216432-medication

[50] Alloubi I. Thoracic hydatid cyst: Clinical presentation, radiological features and surgical treatment. In: Principles and Practice of Cardiothoracic Surgery. IntechOpen; 2013. pp. 195-217

[51] Brunetti E, Filice C. Echinococcosis hydatid cyst. Medicine. 2007:1-23

[52] Cobzaru RG, Popa GT. Historical aspects regarding the regarding the hydatic disease. Section: Social Sciences, Psychology, Sociology and Education Sciences. 2016;**16**(7):103-107

[53] Ekim M, Yılmaz H, Ekim H, Tuncer M, Ozdemir Z. Importance of laboratory tests in the diagnosis and follow up of patients with intrathoracic hydatidosis. Journal of International Research in Medical and Pharmaceutical Sciences. 2016;**6**(2):57-62

[54] Albadawi AAM. Molecular and serological studies on cystic hydatid infection in man and camels in Sudan [PhD thesis]. Sudan University of Science and Technology; 2017

[55] Song XH, Ding LW, Wen H. Bone hydatid disease. Postgraduate Medical Journal. 2007;**83**(982):536-542

[56] Al-Khafaji AMAR. Study of pathological and biochemical changes of cyst disease in humans, sheep and cows in Al-Diwaniya city [master thesis]. College of Veterinary Medicine, University of Al-Qadisiyah; 2006

[57] Eckert J, Deplazes P. Biological, epidemiological and clinical aspects of echinococcosis a zoonosis of increasing concern. Clinical Microbiology. 2004;**17**(1):107-135

[58] Eddi C, de Katalin B, Juan L, William A, Andrew S, Daniela B, et al. Veterinary public health activities at FAO: Cysticercosis and echinococcosis. Parasitology International. 2006;(55):305-308

Section 4

Diagnosis

Chapter 5

Imaging in Echinococcosis

Tuba Apaydın

Abstract

Hydatid disease is a widely common parasitic disease caused by the species; *Echinococcus granulosus* and *Echinococcus multilocularis*. Echinococcosis is a serious medical, economical and social handicap all over the world. Almost any organ of the body can be involved with the zoonosis, liver and lungs are the most frequently involved organs. Imaging has a critical role for diagnosis of the disease. Radiography is the first imaging tool. Although CT aids the detection of size, number, location and imaging of local complications for diagnosis of hydatid cysts, sometimes atypical lesions rise in the imaging tools. MRI may help for differentiation of hydatid lesions from other neoplastic and hypodense infective lesions. MRI is also better for biliary and neurological involvement. Ultrasound is especially helpful for abdominal hydatidosis and peripheral lung lesions. Regarding that clinical evaluation is difficult for hydatidosis; radiological findings should be evaluated well for accurate diagnosis. This chapter will focus on imaging of echinococcosis.

Keywords: *Echinococcus*, MRI, CT, USG, hydatid cyst

1. Introduction

Hydatid disease is a worldwide parasitic infection created by larval phase of *Echinococcus* [1]. Human infection is frequently seen in Europe, Middle East, some places of Canada, Russia, Japan, China, Australia and New Zealand [2].

In the life period, *E. granulosus* stands in the small bowel of its definitive host; carnivores, which are generally dogs and wolves [3]. Then, eggs passed into the feces are ingested with the intermediate host, which is generally sheep [4]. Larval stage occurs in the intermediate host; i.e., ingested eggs outgrows in the small intestine and lets out oncosphere, which invades the intestinal mucosa and come in the lungs, liver or other organs (metacestode larvae). Eggs can survive up to 1 year in the environment. On the next step, definitive host digests the infected organs of the intermediate host. Protoscolices invades the intestinal mucosa and grow up to adult worms [3]. Human being can be more commonly infected by indirect ingestion of contaminated water and food or directly from contact with dogs [4].

Fluid filled cyst is covered with three layers; pericyst, ectocyst and endocyst [5]. Pericyst is created by the protective reaction of the host tissue; the middle laminated layer called ectocyst lets for the transition of nutrients and the germinal layer inside called endocyst generates cyst fluid, blood capsules, scolices and also provides the constitution of ectocyst [5, 6]. Many daughter vesicles remain in the hydatid cysts [6].

Liver is the most commonly affected organ, second one is the lung. Other organs are less commonly affected. Heart is rarely affected, but it's fatal if it's affected. Left ventricule is more commonly affected than the right ventricle possibly due to its richer blood supply. Additionally, huger myocardial mass in left ventricle supplies better circumstances for parasite's growth. Hydatid cysts of left ventricle are generally located in the subepicardium. Rupture into the pericardial space is seldom. However, habitation in the right ventricle is subendocardial, rupture is more common which results with anaphylaxis, pulmonary embolisation and death [7].

Most common way for myocardial invasion is coronary circulation. Second most common route is pulmonary venous drainage with the rupture of pulmonary cysts. Heart may also be involved with direct contact [7].

Hydatid disease has an evolutionary period; first, cysts grow slowly; then, a differentiation period starts which the parasite dies and forms calcified, solidified cyst behind [7].

The lungs are the most common organ in pediatric patients and the second most common organ for adults. Due to the negative pressure inside the lungs, cysts grow three times faster compared to the growth in the liver [6].

E. granulosus has a broad genetic diversity. Molecular gene analysis has defined 10 genotypes, which are aggregated into four different types: *E. granulosus* sensu strict [G1-G3 complex], *Echinococcus equinus* [G4], *Echinococcus ortleppi* [G5] and *Echinococcus canadensis* [G6-G10 complex]. G1 genotype of *E. granulosus* is reported to infect humans more frequently compared to other subtypes. Genotyping of human CE can help to plan the controlling methods for human hydatidosis. Genetic subtyping also clarifies the diversity in development, antigenicity and response to chemotherapeutic agents [3].

The disease is asymptomatic in the inception and can remain asymptomatic for long years even though the cysts become very huge [1]. For symptomatic patients, symptoms appertain to localization of the cyst. Cough, dyspnea or chest pain can be seen if the cysts are in the lung. Abdominal pain, hepatomegaly, sensibility, fever and icterus are the symptoms for liver cysts. With the rupture of the cyst due to the surgical intervention to the cyst or mechanical trauma, patients are prone to go into anaphylactic shock [1]. Cyst rupture can realise throughout the bronchus and patients can present with cough and sputum with hydatid sand and membrane fragments. If the cyst rupture realises throughout the pleural cavity, patients can present with pneumothorax, effusion and emphysema [6]. If the cyst rupture through vena cava, patient can present with recurrent pulmonary embolism [6].

Cysts and cyst like hypodense lesions carry diagnostic debate on computed tomography (CT) in some cases. Tumors with cystic degeneration, inauspicious lesions like necrotic lung cancer, metastases and infections like tuberculosis can imitate hydatid cyst [8].

Diagnosis is quite elementary for hydatid cyst (HC) if typical findings like crescent sign, onion peel, combo sign or folded membranes are present. However, atypical findings like solid or more hypodense semblance of ruptured, collapsed or infected cysts are more complicated as they resemble infections like tuberculosis or neoplastic lesions. MRI may help for diagnosis in these conditions [8]. Ultrasound can help to diagnose peripheral lesions and to achieve pleura [6].

2. Imaging in echinococcosis

Imaging tools for hydatid disease are computed tomography (CT), ultrasonography (USG), magnetic resonance imaging (MRI), radiography and urography.

2.1 Radiography

Radiograph is the primary method for imaging in bone and lung disease. An uncomplicated hydatid cyst looks like a well-limited homogenous radio-opacity on chest X-ray (**Figure 1A**). Cysts quietly resemble carom balls in posteroanterior X-ray and to rugger balls in lateral X-ray [6]. Cysts may look like a strange shaped mass due to pressure of mediastinum, bronchovascular components. Multiple large cysts are also pathognomonic for echinococcosis (**Figure 1B**) [1]. Cysts can present with bilobed appearance due to nicking inside the cysts [6]. The loss of a round shape with a small depressed view points out bronchial rupture, so called "slit sign".

Atelectatic and reactive reactions can result with the loss of well limited borders, thus imitating carcinoma or pneumonia [6].

A radiolucent frame may be seen with the entry of air between pericyst and endocyst due to disruption of bronchus, so called "crescent sign" (**Figure 2**). This sign is not pathognomonic for hydatid cysts and may also be seen in carcinoma, blood clots, mycetoma, and Rasmussen aneurysm. If the entry of air increases, endocyst minimizes and ruptures; an air fluid level is observed in the endocyst, so-called "double curve sign". The natant membranes in the cyst fluid compose "water-lily sign" if there is furthermore collapse of the endocyst. Daughter cysts may look like circular radio-opacities at deep part of the cysts, so-called "rising sun" image. Pericyst can become empty if the membranes are extracted with cough, air-filled cysts can be seen on X-ray, so-called "dry cyst sign". In cases of infection added to the disorder, lung abscess can be imitated (**Figure 3**).

X-rays for abdomen may present with hepatomegaly, elevation of right hemidiaphragm and cyst wall calcification. During healing period of the cyst, all the structures in the cyst calcify and plain radiograph presents a dense calcified mass [5].

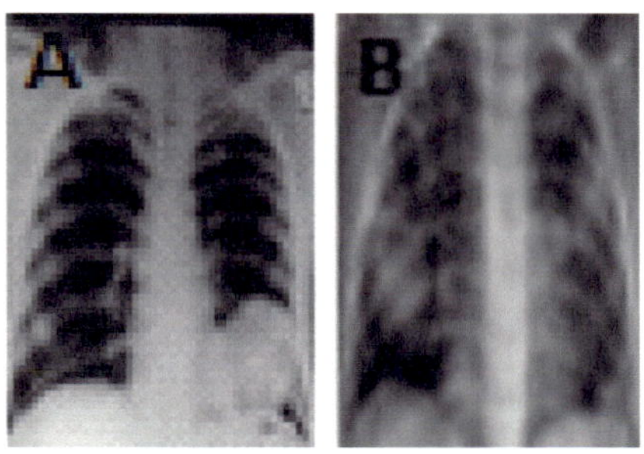

Figure 1.
(A) Posteroanterior view of chest X-ray presenting uncomplicated hydatid cyst of left lower lung and (B) posteroanterior view of chest X-ray presenting multiple, large, circular and well limited masses in both hemithoraces.

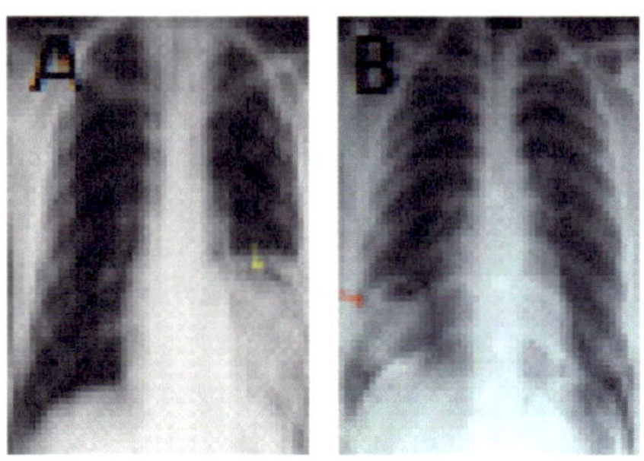

Figure 2.
(A) Chest X-ray showing pulmonary meniscus sign (arrow) indicating crescent shaped containment of air and (B) chest X-ray presenting a well limited lesion (arrow) in the right lower lobe of the lung with air fluid level, indicating a superimposed infection.

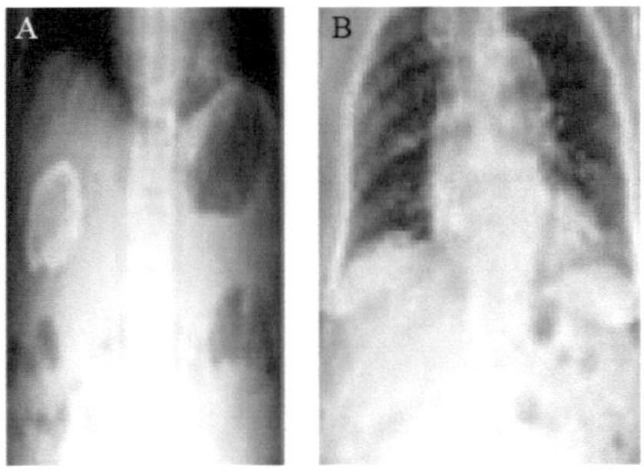

Figure 3.
(A) Abdominal X-ray showing round calcified mass in the right hypochondrium and (B) chest radiograph showing hydatid cyst in the liver.

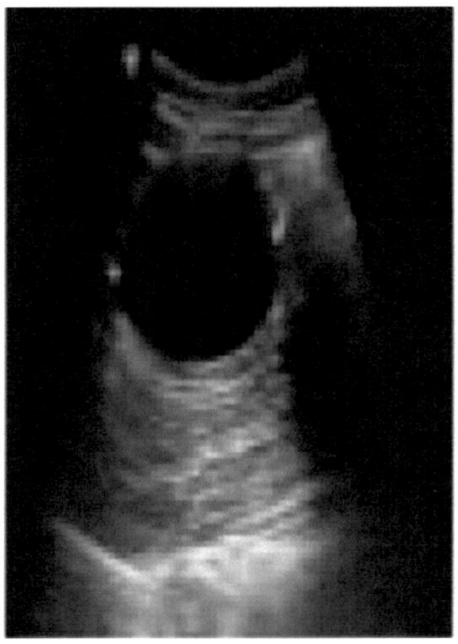

Figure 4.
Transverse ultrasound of the retroperitoneum showing unilocular anechoic cyst (type CL according to WHO classification).

2.2 CT and ultrasonography in hydatid cysts

Cysts don't always present classical signs above. Obstacles about diagnosis can be overlapped with the help of CT in required cases [6]. CT is a significant diagnostic tool in detecting cyst wall or septal calcification, osseous lesions, cystic component localized posterior to calcification, evaluating complications and in cases which USG is not enough (abdominal wall deformities, excessive bowel gases, obesity and previous surgery) [4].

US is easily accessible and lacks radiation. It's sensitivity is about 100% acquiring it the priority as a screening method for abdominal hydatidosis. USG and MRI are both successful to show hydatid sand, daughter cysts, natant membranes and vesicles inside the cyst (**Figure 4**) [1, 4].

Mobile hydatid sand which points out to the splitted capsules and scolices that moves in the cyst cavity may be presented in a "snowstorm" appearance (**Figure 5**). Most commonly used classifications related to sonographic appearance are classifications of Gharbi et al. (**Table 2**) and the World Health Organisation Informal Working Group classification on echinococcosis (WHO-IWGE) (**Table 3**) [5].

Gharbi type 1 is the most common subtype and it's presented as a pure cystic lesion with or without the entity of hydatid sand (**Figures 4** and **5**). Gharbi type II cysts grows out after trauma, cyst degeneration, host response or drug therapy. Decrease in the

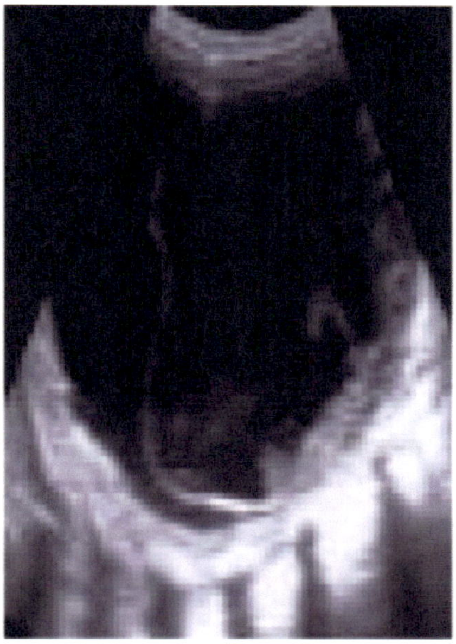

Figure 5.
Longitudinal ultrasound of a liver hydatid cyst in a 8 years old girl presenting the "snowstorm appearance".

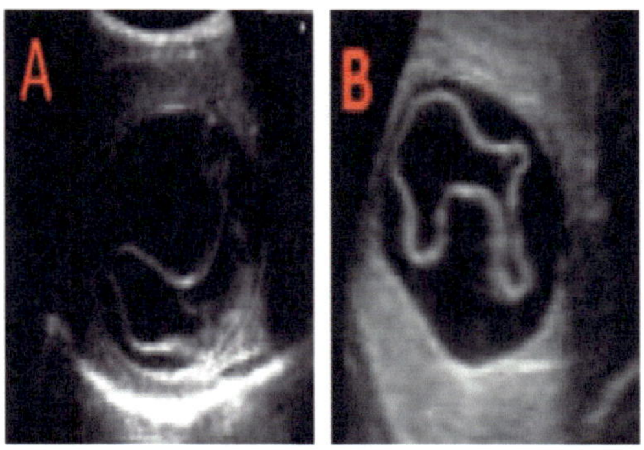

Figure 6.
Ultrasonographic view of Gharbi type II hydatid cysts: (A) "Split wall" sign from splitting of pericyst and endocyst and (B) "water-lily" sign resulting from complete splitting of the membranes.

intracystic pressure results with splitting of the endocyst and pericyst; natant membranes may be seen in the cyst cavity. Complete splitting of the membranes is called as "water-lily" sign due to its morphological appearance (**Figure 6**). Gharbi type III cysts are multivesicular cysts which septae presenting the neighbour borders of daughter cysts composes a "honeycomb" image (**Figure 7**). "Spoke wheel" appearance may be seen when daughter cysts are splitted with hydatid matrix. Gharbi type IV cysts are composed of an internal echogenic matrix giving them a solid appearance (**Figure 8**). For differential diagnosis, daughter cysts or membranes should be searched to externalize a solid mass. Gharbi type V cysts involve wall calcification and dense distal acoustic shadowing (**Figure 9**). A densely calcified cyst can be supposed to be dead. However, a partially calcified cyst should still be regarded as an alive cyst [5].

Imaging findings for hydatid cyst differentiate from cystic lesions to solid appearing lesions. The cyst may look like a well identified fluid accumulation. There may be the appearance of natant membranes due to cleavage of endocyst from pericyst. Ring like calcification of the cyst can lead to complete calcification during differentiation of the cyst [2].

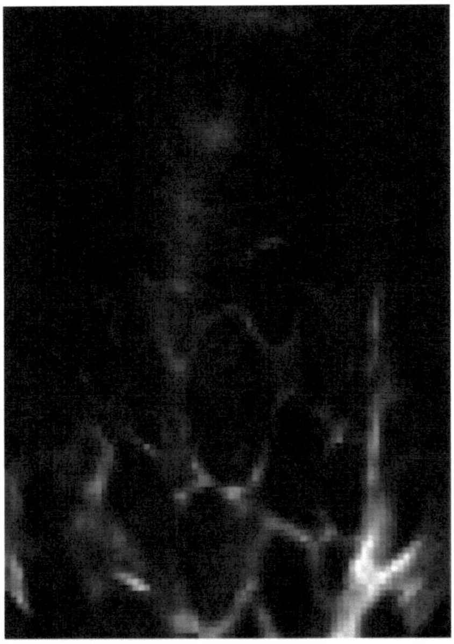

Figure 7.
Transverse ultrasound of Gharbi type III hydatid cyst of liver multiple daughter cysts in an echogenic matrix results in a "honeycomb" image.

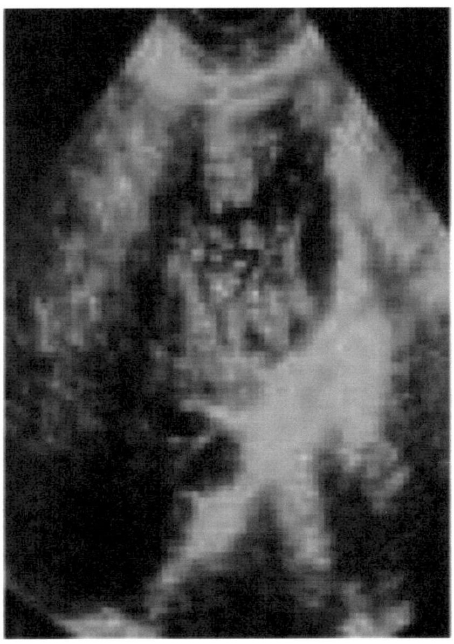

Figure 8.
Ultrasonographic appearance of Gharbi type IV hydatid cyst of the liver.

Specific findings of imaging are visualization of daughter cysts, calcification of the cyst wall and membrane detachment. Diagnosis in early stage is hard [1].

Appearance of hydatid disease may be classified into four subtypes.

Type I is simple cyst with no internal tectonic. On ultrasound, type 1 hydatid cysts seem as well identified unilocular anechoic lesions (**Figure 10**). On CT, they seem as fluid accumulated lesions. MRI demonstrates a fluid accumulated cystic lesion with a T1 isointense and T2 hypointense peripheral border (rim sign) enclosing the homogenous high signal cyst ingredients [2].

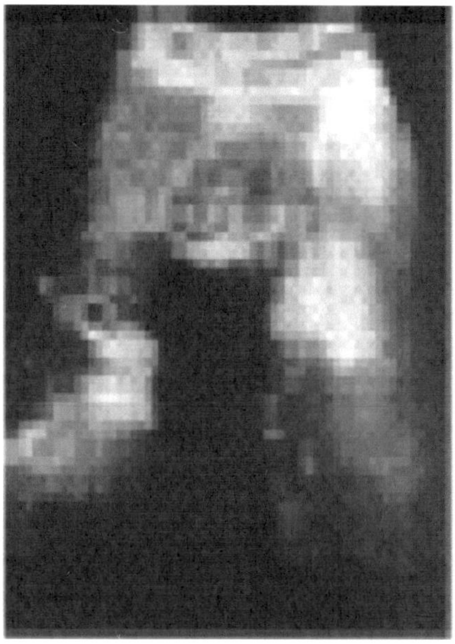

Figure 9.
Ultrasonographic appearance of Gharbi type V hydatid cyst.

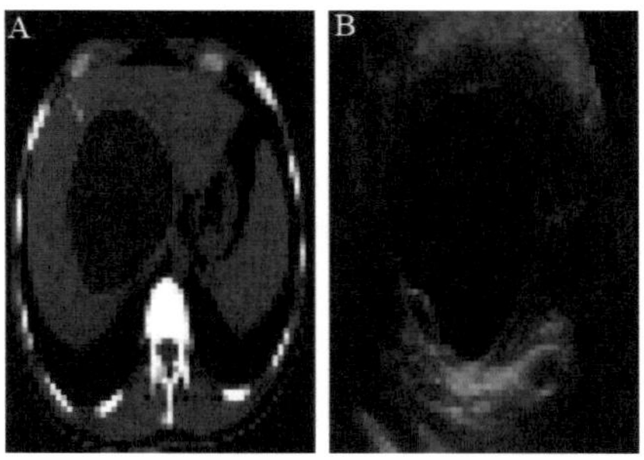

Figure 10.
Type 1 hydatid cyst: (A) axial contrast CT image of a 15 years old female presents a well identified fluid accumulated simple cystic lesion in the liver and (B) oblique sonogram in a 45 years old male demonstrates type 1 hydatid cyst in the liver.

Type II hydatid cysts are cysts with daughter cysts and matrix. They include cleaved natant membranes or daughter cysts (**Figure 11**). Attenuation of the daughter cyst is hypodense/hypointense to maternal matrix on CT and MRI, respectively. If there are multiple cysts, they are covered with a single capsule presenting with a "truckle spoke" appearance [2].

Type II HC are classified to three subtypes according to the age, quantity and setting of the daughter cysts.

Type IIa contain involve daughter cysts organized at the periphery.

Type IIb involve bigger daughter cysts with irregular borders that covers almost all of the capacity of the mother cyst.

Type IIc contains high attenuation round or oval masses with sprinkled calcifications and daughter cysts, demonstrating attrition of the old cyst.

Type III cysts are dead calcified cysts (**Figure 12**).

Type IV hydatid cysts are complicated cysts (**Figure 13**). Most common complications of echinococcosis are rupture and superinfection. Degeneration of parasitic membranes causes the rupture of the cyst (**Figures 14–18**).

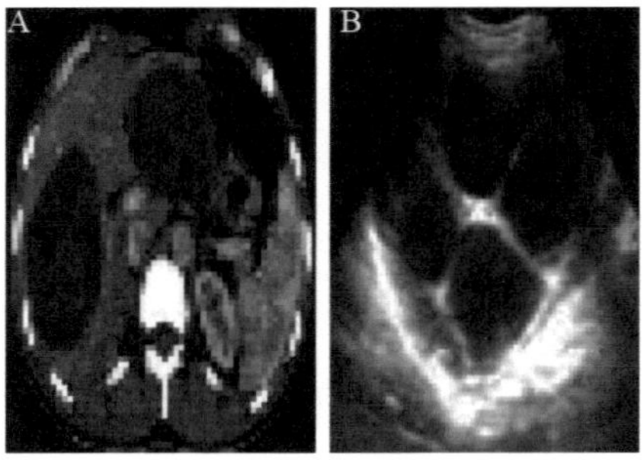

Figure 11.
Type 2 hydatid cyst: (A) contrast enhanced computed tomography demonstrates multiple daughter cysts with irregular borders covering almost all of the volume of the mother cyst-so called "rosette appearance" and (B) oblique ultrasonogram in a 39 years old male demonstrates type 2 hydatid cyst.

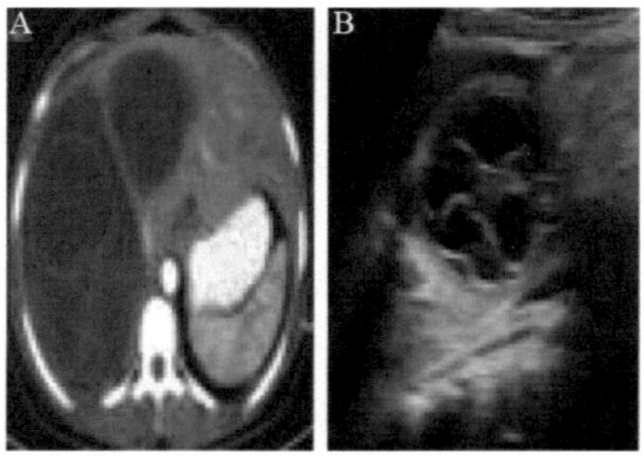

Figure 12.
Type 3 hydatid cyst: (A) contrast enhanced computed tomography presents type 3 hydatid cyst in the right lobe of the liver and (B) oblique ultrasonogram shows anechoic lesion with membranes floating on the cyst fluid.

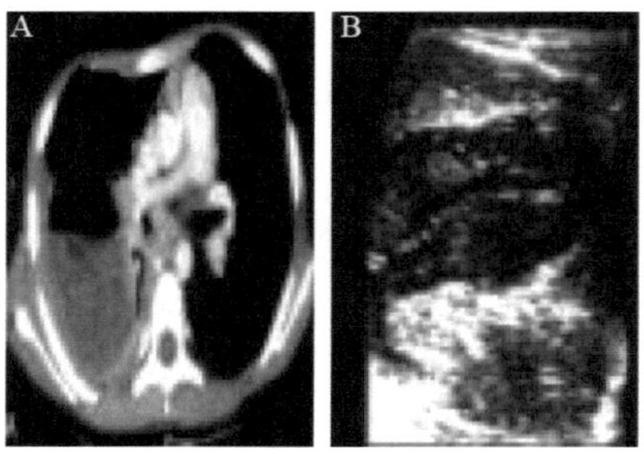

Figure 13.
Type 4 hydatid cyst: (A) sagittal contrast enhanced CT images of thorax show ruptured type 4 hydatid cyst in the lower lobe of the right lung with wrinkled floating endocyst-so called "lily sign" and (B) oblique ultrasonogram shows type 4 hydatid cyst.

Various secondary complications possibly happen according to site of rupture in the body. Secondary complications of echinococcosis according to different locations are listed in **Table 1**.

Gharbi et al. preferred classification for differentiation of subtypes of hydatid cysts on ultrasonogram of the liver (**Table 1**) [5].

Another global classification used for sonographic imaging of hydatid cysts wad presented by World Health Organization Informal Working Group (**Table 2**) [5].

Type	Description
Type I	Pure fluid accumulation
Type II	Fluid accumulation with splitted membrane
Type III	Fluid accumulation with septa and/or daughter cysts
Type IV	Heterogenous echo pattern (hyperechoic with high internal echoes)
Type V	Cyst with calcified thick borders

Table 1.
Gharbi et al. classification of hydatid cysts related to ultrasonographic features [5].

Type	Description
Type CL	Unilocular, cystic lesions with uniform anechoic ingredient, not absolutely confined with hyperechoic frame.
Type CE1	Unilocular, simple cyst with uniform anechoic ingredient. Cyst can present with echoes because of moving capsules, so called ''hydatid sand''(flack sign)
Type CE2	Multivesicular and multiseptated cysts; cyst septations cause tire like architecture, daughter cysts present ''rosette-like'' or ''honey-comb'' like architecture.
Type CE3	Anechoic ingredient with splitted laminated membrane from the cyst wall seen as natant membrane or as ''waterlily sign'' which points out more membranes natant in the cyst fluid.
Type CE4	This may present with a ''ball of wool'' sign presenting retrograded membranes.
Type CE5	Thick calcified wall of the cyst is belt shaped and produces a cone shaped shadow.

Table 2.
Types of hydatid cysts observed on ultrasound examination of liver [5].

2.3 Magnetic resonance imaging in hydatid cysts

MRI is better to show cyst wall defect, biliary and neurological involvement. Cysts are hyperintense on T2W images and are covered by a low signal frame possibly because of the collagen rich pericyst [1]. If available, daughter cysts are hypointense compared to the intracystic fluid on T1 weighted imaging and hyperintense on T2-weighted images [5]. DW MRI makes the differentiation of CE1 hydatid cysts from other simple cysts with their hyperintense image. Apparent diffusion coefficient (ADC) of the hydatid cyst is lower compared to ADC of simple cyst because of internal viscous contents [1]. Also, ADC values of simple cysts and type I to III hydatid cysts are higher than ADC values of abscesses because diffusion of protons throughout thin fluid is limited. ADC values of type IV hydatid cysts and abscesses present no considerable statistical difference [5].

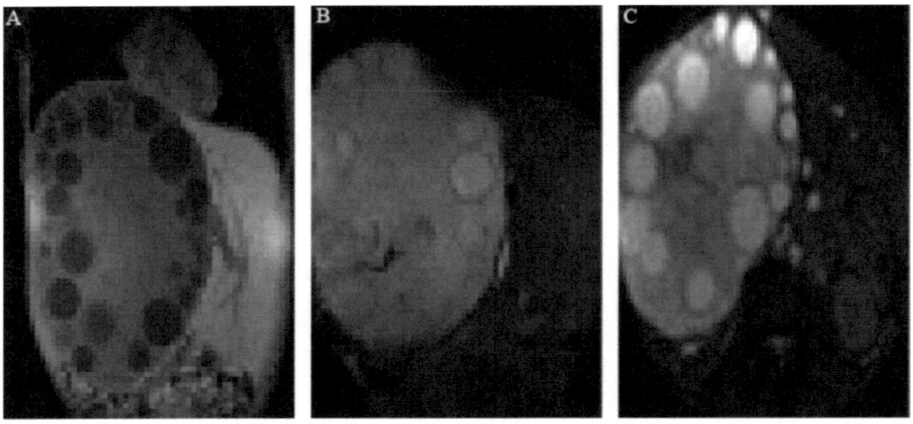

Figure 14.
MRI showing hydatid cyst in the liver of a 45 years old male: (A) coronal T1 weighted image, (B) coronal T2 weighted scan and (C) axial T2 weighted scan.

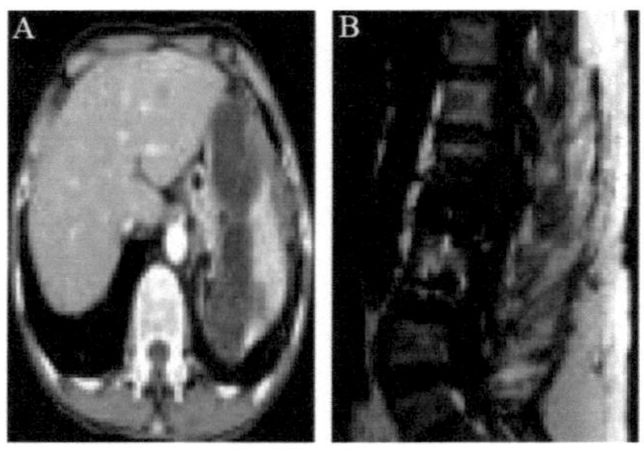

Figure 15.
(A) Axial T2 weighted MRI showing splenic hydatid cyst and (B) coronal T2 weighted scan of hydatid disease in L4-5 vertebra.

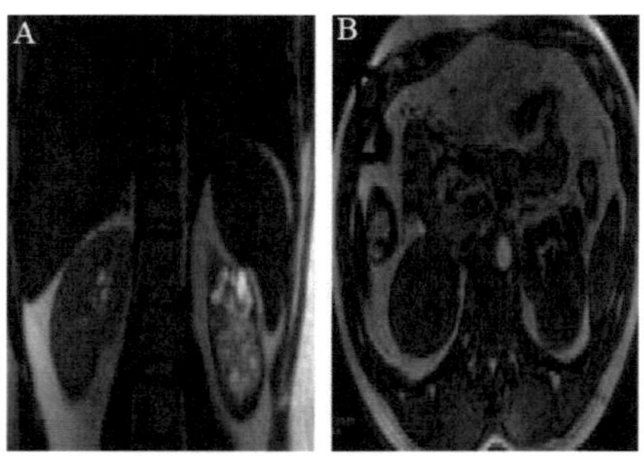

Figure 16.
MRI showing hydatid cyst in the lower pole of the kidney: (A) coronal T1 weighted scan and (B) axial T2 weighted scan.

MRI demonstrates the degree of cyst degeneration with secession of the wall, collapsed membranes are observed as bent linear compositions inside the cyst. Wall calcification is demonstrated better on MRI compared to CT, besides MRI is more successful than CT to represent irregularities of borders that points out inchoative segregation of membranes [5].

MRI is also better to differentiate liver hydatid cysts from other simple cysts [4] (**Figures 14–18**).

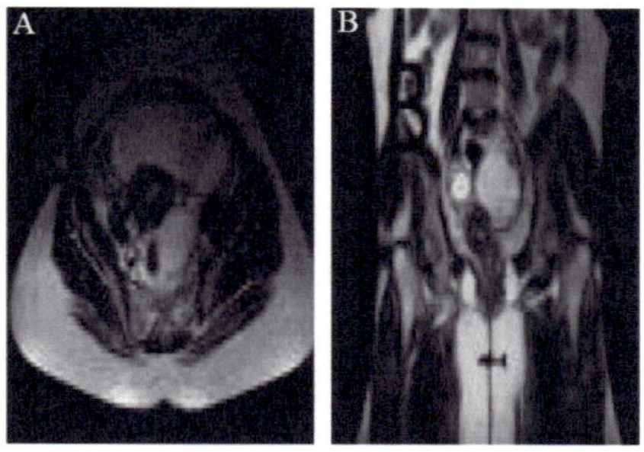

Figure 17.
MRI showing hydatid cyst in the cyst hydatid in the mesosalpinx adjacent to the left ovary: (A) axial T2 weighted image and (B) coronal T2 weighted image.

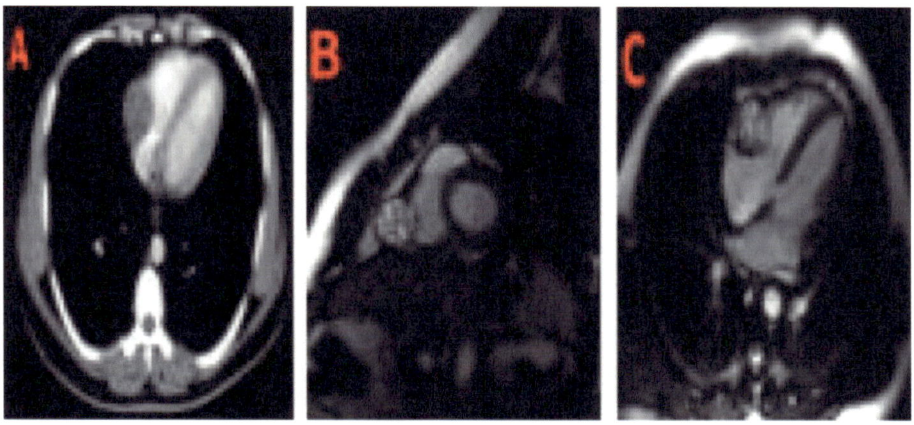

Figure 18.
Case of cardiac cyst hydatid: (A) computed tomographic image, (B) magnetic resonance imaging of transverse section, and (C) magnetic resonance imaging of longitudinal section showing daughter cysts.

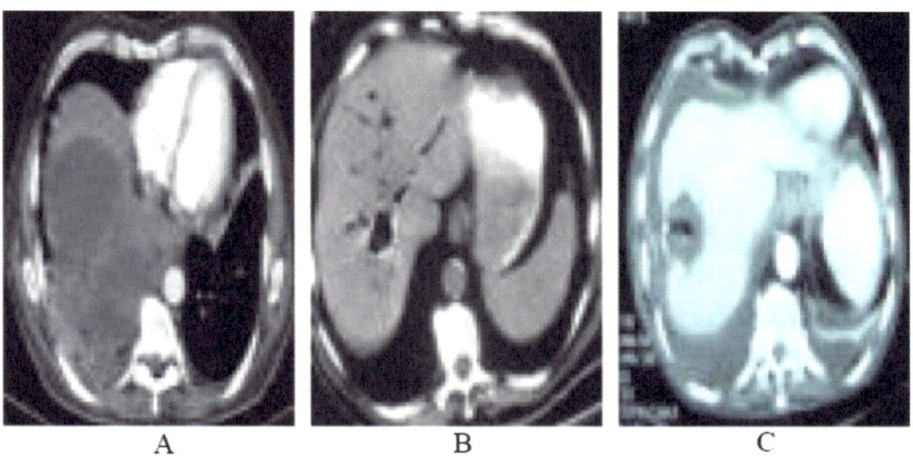

Figure 19.
(A) CT image of rupture of hydatid cyst in the lung, (B) CT scan of intrabiliary rupture of hydatid cyst. (C) CT scan showing intraperitoneal cyst rupture with diffuse peritoneal effusion.

In cardiac cystic echinococcosis, trans-thoracic echocardiography, CT and MRI can demonstrate the cystic structure of the lesion and it's correlation with the cardiac chamber [8] (**Figure 18**).

Location	%	Complications
Liver	71.9	Cyst rupture, liver abcess, inferior vena cava compression and thrombosis, portal hypertension, Budd Chiari syndrome, cholangitis, pancreatitis, biliary peritonitis, peritoneal spread
Lung	19,6	Pneumothorax, lung abcess, biliptysis, lung embolism, pneumonia
Peritoneal &pelvic cavity	3,6	Mass effect
Spleen	2,15	Rupture into peritoneal cavity
Skin&muscles	1,2	Pain, movement disorder
Bones	0,65	Morphologic deformities, pain
Brain	0,56	Seizures, headache, tumor like symptoms

Table 3.
Frequency and location specific complications of hydatid disease [2].

ERCP and MRCP show cystobiliary relationship, daughter vesicles & germinative membranes of cysts in bile ducts, dilated bile ducts. However, because of high intracystic pressure, communication of cyst with bile ducts can't be shown via ERCP& MRCP effectively [1].

2.4 Imaging of complications

Complications like rupture into the peritoneal cavity, biliary cavity and the pleura are presented in **Figure 19**. Incidence and location specific complications of hydatid disease is presented in **Table 3** [2].

3. Conclusion

Echinococcosis is a disorder of larval incursion by echinococcus tapeworm, prevalent in various continents in the world. Lungs and liver are the most commonly affected organs. Imaging has a significant role to implement the right treatment techniques. US is easily accessible and lacks radiation. MRI, CT and ERCP are also used for complicated cases.

Acknowledgements

No contribution by any other author or no funding declared.

Conflict of interest

The authors declare no conflict of interest.

Author details

Tuba Apaydin
Department of Thoracic Surgery, SBU Istanbul Mehmet Akif Ersoy Thoracic and Cardiovascular Training and Research Hospital, Istanbul, Turkey

*Address all correspondence to: tubaapaydn72@gmail.com

References

[1] Devi MA, Venumadhav T, Sukanya B. Role of imaging in diagnosis, predicting biological activity and in treatment plan of hydatid disease. Open Journal of Internal Medicine. 2018;**8**(3):177-195. DOI: 10.4236/ojim.2018.83018

[2] Srinivas MR, Deepashri B, Lakshmeesha MT. Imaging spectrum of hydatid disease: Usual and unusual locations. Polish Journal of Radiology. 2016;**81**:190-205. DOI: 10.12659/PJR.895649

[3] Sarkar M, Pathania R, Jhobta A. Cystic pulmonary hydatidosis. Lung India. 2016;**33**(2):179-191. DOI: 10.4103/0970-2113.177449

[4] Mehta P, Prakash M, Khandelwal N. Radiological manifestations of hydatid disease and its complications. Tropical Parasitology. 2016;**6**(2):103-112. DOI: 10.4103/2229-5070.190812

[5] Banderker E, Cox S, Gaxa L. Imaging and management of abdominal echinococcosis in children. Journal of Pediatric Infectious Diseases. 2017;**12**(01):030-039. DOI: 10.1055/s-0037-1599118

[6] Garg MK, Sharma M, Gulati A. Imaging in pulmonary hydatid cysts. World Journal of Radiology. 2016;**8**(6): 581-587. DOI: 10.4329/wjr.v8.i6.581

[7] Carita P, Verdecchia M, Ferro G. Multimodality imaging in cardiac echinococcosis for diagnosis and follow-up of an untreatable cyst. Internal Journal of Cardiology. 2016;**221**:468-470. DOI: 10.1016/j.ijcard.2016.06.317

[8] Tandur R, Irodi A, Chacko BR. Magnetic resonance imaging as an adjunct to computed tomography in the diagnosis of pulmonary hydatid cysts. Indian Journal of Radiology and Imaging. 2018;**28**(3):342-349. DOI: 10.4103/ijri.IJRI_121_18

Section 5

Treatment

Chapter 6

Medical Treatment of Cystic Echinococcosis

Irina Magdalena Dumitru

Abstract

Medical treatment in cystic echinococcosis is limited; albendazole remains the gold treatment for patients with low hydatid cysts or those with inoperable echinococcosis. Due to uncommon side effects, administration may be continuous (cycles of 28 days with a break of 14 days between courses) as well as discontinuous over long periods of time. In recent years, there have been many concerns for the testing of various substances and drugs against *Echinococcus granulosus*, both in vitro and in vivo, on the animal model, but the results have not been satisfactory. New clinical trials are required, as well as the development of an effective vaccine to limit the spread of echinococcosis in endemic areas.

Keywords: albendazole, hydatid cysts, medical treatment, vaccine, endemic areas

1. Introduction

Treatment of uncomplicated cystic echinococcosis (CE) is complex and consists of medical treatment, surgical and puncture, aspiration, injection, and reaspiration (PAIR), depending on the characteristics of the cyst. For some cases (CE4 and CE5), a conservative "watch and wait" approach is preferred (**Table 1**) [1, 2], because hydatid cysts may spontaneously regress with calcification without chemotherapeutic intervention [3].

Medical treatment has a role in reducing the size of cysts and stopping their development and reducing infectivity and is the only therapeutic option in inoperable cases. The combination of medical treatment with surgery (preoperative and postoperative administration) or PAIR plays a role in preventing recurrences [4].

2. The current state of knowledge

Mebendazole (MBZ) was the initial agent, but it has proven less effective than albendazole over time (10–15 mg/kg/day, maximum 800 mg orally in two doses) [5]. Because MBZ is insoluble in water and has a poor solubility and bioavailability, the drug is poorly effective [5]. The recommended regimen is 40–50 mg/kg/day, orally in three divided doses during meals, in long-term therapy (more than 2 years), and the success rate is 14–49% of cases [1]. MBZ is more effective in small cysts <5 cm in size, and the therapeutic response was superior in pulmonary (83%) than in hepatic (18%) locations [6]. MBZ treatment is well tolerated in long term therapy; adverse events have been described in 5–40% of patients—gastrointestinal distress, hair loss, neutropenia, anaphylactic reactions, glomerulonephritis, vertigo,

WHO classification	Suggested practice
CE1	Albendazole alone if <5 cm PAIR + albendazole if >5 cm
CE2	Surgery + albendazole or Non-PAIR PT + albendazole
CE3a	Albendazole alone if <5 cm PAIR + albendazole if >5 cm
CE3b	Surgery + albendazole Non-PAIR PT + albendazole
CE4 and CE5	Wait and watch

Table 1.
Treatment modalities stratified by cyst stage [1].

headache, psychic conspicuousness, hematotoxic effects, and abnormal levels of serum transaminases [7]—and so MBZ treatment is not recommended in pregnant women during the first trimester of pregnancy because it is associated with congenital abnormalities of the fetus [8].

The standard regimen of albendazole (ABZ) is cycles of 28 days with a break of 14 days between courses, but duration of treatment is different depending on many factors.

Velasco-Tirado et al. show that in a meta-analysis performed on 33 cystic echinococcosis treatment-related studies, there are insufficient data to standardize the results, and the optimal duration of therapy has not yet been established [9].

A study conducted by Dumitru et al., in Constanta, Romania, on 320 patients diagnosed with hydatid cyst, during 5 years (2008–2013), showed that six therapeutic cures were necessary before the first healing signs appeared [10] in most of cases and the response to treatment depends on the location of the cyst, size, and type according to Gharbi classification and immune status.

Related to location, albendazole treatment's efficiency is higher in the case of hepatic or pulmonary localization than in other localizations (7.428571 ± 1.886039 cures) [11]. Dimension <7 cm (especially <5 cm) responds better to medical treatment, and the number of therapeutic cures administered for the CE1 (6.739 ± 1.91 cures) is significantly smaller than the number of cures administered for the CE3 (8.181 ± 2.39 cures) [11]. Long-term treatment with albendazole (more than 6 months) was only used for multiple or inoperable CE [11].

In the same study, we concluded that patients with good immune status responded better to albendazole treatment than to patients with CD4 < 500 cells/mm^3; also, the presence of comorbidities such as diabetes and chronic hepatitis was a negative predictive factor [11].

An additional study, conducted by the same team on a group of HIV-infected patients diagnosed with CE, with low CD4 (<200 cells/mm^3), demonstrated that continuous therapy with albendazole 800 mg/day, administered more than 6 months, was not effective, and CD4 count can be a predictive factor for response to medical treatment [12].

Preoperative treatment with albendazole begins 1–3 months (average 14 days) before surgery and/or PAIR and continues for 1–3 months posttreatment [1, 3].

Because absorption of albendazole in humans is very variable, it is considered that concomitant administration of fatty meal would increase the absorption [13].

In recent years, the occurrence of resistance to albendazole has been frequently discussed, which greatly limits the medical treatment of echinococcosis [14]. Recent study conducted by Mortezaei et al. has shown that genetic makeup and miRNA profile of helminths affect their response to albendazole sulfoxide (ABZ-SOX) and revealed significant differential expression of let-7 and miR-61 at different drug concentrations [14]. This may explain the poor response to ABZ-SOX in some patients and requires the emergence of more effective new therapies.

A large meta-analysis conducted on 711 patients from 5 countries shows that multivesicular, multi-septated, and transitional cysts responded poorly to benzimidazoles (BMZ) and were associated to a high rate of relapses and BMZ are effective only in small cysts (diameter < 6 cm) [4]. Other factors that influence the response to therapy with benzimidazoles are age, because young patients respond much better to treatment than older people, and on the other hand, cyst localization influences the response to treatment; bone cysts were less susceptible to BMZ than hepatic or pulmonary echinococcosis [11, 15].

Albendazole long therapy is well tolerated; therefore, many clinicians prefer continuous therapy more than discontinuous therapy.

Because ABZ is nowadays considered a relatively safe drug, continuous therapy is preferred over discontinuous treatment protocols. The reported side effects were more frequent hepatotoxicity, alopecia, and gastrointestinal disturbances and less common jaundice, severe headache, cough, jaundice, vertigo, and itching [16]. ABZ is embryotoxic and teratogenic in pregnant women [17].

Recent studies have shown that concomitant administration of ABZ with certain drugs has a synergistic effect. Adding metformin to classical treatment with ABZ (an antidiabetic drug) has increased the efficacy of ABZ in vitro and in vivo (mouse models) [18, 19]. ABZ-mefloquine combined treatment seems a promising combination, with results slightly superior to monotherapy with ABZ [20].

In recent years, researchers' efforts have focused on new ABZ formulations that lead to better tissue and organ penetration, including liposomes, biodegradable microspheres, and polymer conjugates. In this manner the drug is released for prolonged periods of time, improving the therapeutic effect [21].

Praziquantel (PZQ) is a less effective antiparasitic drug than albendazole in the treatment of CE but in combination with ABZ might be helpful than ABZ alone in disseminated and inoperable cases [22, 23]. PZQ 40 mg/kg once a week in combination with ABZ 800 mg/day has proven more effective than ABZ alone, both before surgical intervention or PAIR and in the treatment of inoperable cases [23, 24]. Also, a combined therapy with ABZ 10 mg/kg/day and PZQ 25 mg/kg/day is effective as a prophylactic, preoperative treatment [25].

Isolated studies have demonstrated the antiparasitic properties of some drugs in vivo or only in vitro, but all studies have concluded that there is no alternative drug to albendazole to treat echinococcosis and it needs more research to discover new drugs [26, 27].

- **Ursodeoxycholic acid** had some scolicidal effects and can be administered to patients with poor response to albendazole therapy, in combination [28].

- ***Lawsonia inermis*** and ***Achillea millefolium*** **extracts** are a potent protoscolicidal which may be used as a scolicidal agent during the surgery. *Achillea millefolium* extracts at the concentration of 3 mg/ml after 5 minutes of exposure killed all of the protoscolices, and *Lawsonia inermis* extracts at concentration of 3 mg/ml after 10 minutes of exposure killed also all the protoscolices [28].

- **Sodium arsenite (NaAsO2)** administered in combination with albendazole significantly increases sensitivity of *Echinococcus granulosus* protoscoleces to ABZ, and the maximum protoscolicidal effect was seen with the combination 20 μM NaAsO2 + 80 μM ABZ [29].

- **Garlic chloroformic extract** had high protoscolicidal effects in recent study conducted by Barzin et al. in 2019 and could substitute other agents. The study compared the effectiveness of garlic extract with sodium chloride and silver nitrate and demonstrated that the protoscolicidal effects of the garlic extract at 1 ($P < 0.001$) and 2 ($P < 0.001$ and $P = 0.003$) minutes of exposure were higher than those of sodium chloride and silver nitrate. At 5 minutes of exposure, there was no difference between the garlic extract and sodium chloride ($P = 0.36$) [30].

- Anti-theilerial drugs **MMV689480 (buparvaquone)** and **MMV671636 (ELQ-400)** have demonstrated a cytotoxic effect [29]. Buparvaquone impaired parasite mitochondria, and with an IC50 of 2.87 μM and 0.02 μM, respectively, against in vitro cultured *E. multilocularis* metacestodes, buparvaquone can be an effective therapeutic choice [31].

- *Myrtus communis* methanolic extract and ***Tripleurospermum disciforme*** have proven a scolicidal effect [30]. They can be used during hydatid surgery and could prevent the secondary infection. The results indicated that the highest scolicidal effect (100%) of *M. communis* was obtained at 100 and 50 mg/ml concentrations and LC50 in 10, 20, and 30 minutes were 11.64, 7.62, and 6.47 mg/ml, respectively. Further studies are required for identification of the active ingredients in the extracts [32].

- **Chitosan nanoparticles containing curcumin (Ch-Cu NPs)** had a good activity against *Echinococcus granulosus* in study published by Napooni et al. and can be considered an anti-protoscolex agent [33].

- **Mebendazole C1 (M-C1)** and **mebendazole C2 (M-C2)**, two isoforms obtained from the reaction of mebendazole with epichlorohydrin, have superior efficacy on *Echinococcus multilocularis* protoscoleces and metacestodes compared to mebendazole [34]. It was also found that the introduction of an epoxy group to mebendazole reduced its cytotoxicity in rat hepatoma (RH) cells. The conclusion of the study was that introduction of an epoxy group to mebendazole improved the solubility of mebendazole, increased the parasiticidal effects on *E. multilocularis*, and reduced its cytotoxicity in RH cells [34].

- **Anacardic acid (AA)** is a natural product isolated from the Brazilian cashew-nut shell liquid and presented a high activity against metacestodes of *Echinococcus multilocularis* (*E. multilocularis*) and *Echinococcus granulosus sensu stricto* (*E. granulosus* s.s.) in vitro and in vivo [35]. Yuan et al. demonstrated that anacardic acid (AA) has better efficacy than albendazole (ABZ) in vitro against Echinococcus metacestode and has similar efficacy to albendazole in vivo and the researchers concluded that AA may be an effective anti-*Echinococcus* drug in the future [36].

- **Pentamidine** (MMV000062), **alpha-difluoromethylornithine** (MMV001625), and **suramin** (MMV637953) were all tested in vivo against *E. granulosus*, but did not show any effects [36, 37].

- **Rifampicin** (MMV688775) and **miltefosine** (MMV688990) were ineffective in vivo against *E. granulosus* [36, 38].

- **Amphotericin B** (MMV689000) which is an antifungal drug has demonstrated a good activity against *E. multilocularis* metacestodes in vitro at 2.7 μM [39–41]. Reiter et al. concluded that in some cases, amphotericin B therapy may be a salvage treatment in patients with progressive human alveolar echinococcosis [39] but is considered a limited therapy and is administered to well-selected patients due to increased nephrotoxicity [40, 42].

- **Nitazoxanide** (MMV688991) has been studied by Stettler et al. who demonstrated that it has a good activity against *E. granulosus* metacestodes and protoscoleces in vitro [43–46]. Nitazoxanide was also tested in vivo in mice and in human patients with cystic (CE) and alveolar (AE) echinococcosis, but no beneficial effects were observed compared to ABZ [43–46].

- **Auranofin** (MMV688978) is a thioredoxin-glutathione reductase inhibitor and has the property of killing *E. granulosus* protoscoleces and is also active against *E. multilocularis* metacestodes [47, 48]. The studies reported a good efficacy in vitro at 2.5 μM after 48 h [49, 50].

- **Mefloquine** (MMV000016) is an antiparasitic drug used in malaria, active on *Plasmodium* spp., which has proven to be effective against *Echinococcus multilocularis* metacestodes in vitro and in vivo [51–54]. In a study conducted by Küster (2011), oral administration of mefloquine (25 mg/kg of body weight administered twice a week for a period of 8 weeks) was compared with albendazole (200 mg/kg/day) or mefloquine intraperitoneally compared with albendazole. The study was performed on mice infected with *Echinococcus multilocularis* and showed similar efficacy of mefloquine administered intraperitoneally, compared to oral albendazole [52]. Oral administration of mefloquine at higher doses and over a long period of time (200 mg/kg, 5 days per week, during 4 weeks followed by treatments of 100 mg/kg during the last 7 weeks) had superior efficacy [53].

- **Pomegranate peel aqueous extract** (PGE) in combination with albendazole has anti-hydating and anti-inflammatory effects in vivo, in mice infected with *Echinococcus granulosus* [55]. The researchers consider that PGE has a significant additive anti-hydatid effect and is beneficial in the preventive treatment of recurrences [55].

- ***Pelargonium roseum*** and *Ferula gummosa* are essential oils with scolicidal properties, without side effect [56]. Tabari et al. have shown that protoscoleces of *E. granulosus* have a high potential against their two main constituents, citronellol and β-pinene, and toxic effect on *E. granulosus* in intraoperative use in hydatid cyst patients.

- BMZ analogs like **fenbendazole, flubendazole, oxfendazole**, and **triclabendazole** have been evaluated in the last years, in vitro and in vivo studies (animal models), but did not provide superior efficacy compared to mebendazole or albendazole [57].

- **Ivermectin** is an antiparasitic drug which is used against nematodes and has scolicidal activity if injected directly into the cyst during laparoscopy in a rodent but has a poor activity if administered orally due to low cyst penetration [58].

- **Cyclosporine A** is an immunosuppressant drug and described scolicidal activity in vitro and can be used for pre- and posttreatment in surgery or aspiration techniques [59].

- **Imatinib and pyridinylimidazoles** (anti-neoplastic drugs, kinase inhibitors) show therapeutic effects on the parasite, both in vitro and in vivo, on the animal model [60].

- Natural compounds like **thymol, menthol, and plant extracts** (*Trachyspermum ammi* L. fruit essential oil, *Zataria* multiflora and *Origanum vulgare* essential oils, *Salvia officinalis*, *Mentha* spp. essential oil, *Rosmarinus officinalis* essential oil, *Allium sativum* methanol or chloroform extract, *Berberis vulgaris* aqueous extract, *Cnidium monnieri* osthole, *Corylus* spp., *Curcurbita* spp. hydroalcoholic extracts, *Curcuma longa* ethanol extract, *Mallotus philippinensis* fruit methanol extract, *Nigella sativa* seed essential oil, *Olea europaea* leaves aqueous extract, *Penicillium* extracted chitosan, *Penicillium aculeatum* in silver particles, *Pestalotiopsis* spp. ethyl acetate extract, *Pistacia atlantica* fruit methanol extract, *Punica granatum* peel aqueous extract, *Salvadora persica* root ethanol extract, *Sambucus ebulus* fruit methanol extract, *Satureja khuzestanica* leaves hydroalcoholic extract, *Trametes robiniophila* Murr. aqueous extract, and *Zingiber officinale* ethanol extract) have protoscoleces effects in vitro or in vivo, in different administrations such as oral or intragastric administration [57].

Recent studies have also tried to make albendazole more effective through nanotechnology. Ullio Gamboa et al. have demonstrated that ABZ lipid nanocapsules (ABZ-LNCs) are more effective than ABZ in vivo, in *Echinococcus granulosus* infected mice, in oral administration [61]. These results suggest that ABZ-LNCs could be a promising drug in the treatment of cystic echinococcosis in patients who are poorly responsive or nonresponsive to classical therapy with albendazole.

3. Future directions

In the future, vaccination could prevent the spread of echinococcosis in endemic regions. Zhao et al. identified six dominant T-cell epitopes and five dominant B-cell epitopes in the EgA31 protein structure and six dominant T-cell epitopes and three dominant B-cell epitopes in EgG1Y162 which may represent a beginning for multi-epitope vaccines against *Echinococcus granulosus* [62]. Miles et al. identified 9 novel proteins and 14 peptides to be further tested as potential cystic echinococcosis vaccine candidates [63]. Pilot field trial of the EG95 vaccine against ovine cystic echinococcosis conducted by Larrieu et al. in Argentina demonstrated a decrease in EC incidence and a good surveillance and control tool in the epidemiological chain of the parasite [64].

The development of recombinant bi-vaccines expressing EG95 *Echinococcus granulosus* antigen is a new orientation in the future. Goatpox (GPV) disease and cystic hydatidosis can be prevented by live-attenuated GPV AV41 vaccine; the GPV is an ideal vector for expressing the EG95 antigen [65]. The same group of researchers have developed another recombinant, bivalent vaccine using morbillivirus (SRMV) which expresses EG95 antigen [66], preventing both morbillivirus infection and *Echinococcus granulosus* infection.

Given that treatment in the CE is limited, new clinical trials are needed to find potential drugs and new strategies to limit transmission of infection.

Author details

Irina Magdalena Dumitru
Ovidius University of Constanta, Clinical Infectious Diseases Hospital Constanta, Romania

*Address all correspondence to: dumitrui@hotmail.com

References

[1] Brunetti E, Kern P, Vuitton DA. Writing panel for the WHO-IWGE. Expert consensus for the diagnosis and treatment of cystic and alveolar echinococcosis in humans. Acta Tropica. 2010;**114**(1):1-16

[2] World Health Organization (WHO) Informal Working Group of Echinococcosis. Puncture, Aspiration, Injection, Re-Aspiration. An option for the Treatment of Cystic Echinococcosis. Document WHO/CDS/CSR/SPH/2001.6. Geneva, Switzerland: WHO; 2001. pp. 1-40

[3] De Rosa F, Teggi A. Treatment of *Echinococcus granulosus* hydatid disease with albendazole. Annals of Tropical Medicine and Parasitology. 1990;**84**:467-472

[4] Stojkovic M, Zwahlen M, Teggi A, Vutova K, Cretu CM, Virdone R, et al. Treatment response of cystic Echinococcosis to benzimidazoles: A systematic review. PLoS Neglected Tropical Diseases. 2009;**3**:e524

[5] Davis A, Dixon H, Pawlowski ZS. Multicentre clinical trials of benzimidazole-carbamates in human cystic echinococcosis (phase 2). Bulletin of the World Health Organization. 1989;**67**:503-508

[6] Kern P. Human echinococcosis: Follow-up of 23 patients treated with mebendazole. Infection. 1983;**11**:17-24

[7] Braithwaite PA, Roberts MS, Allan RJ, Watson TR. Clinical pharmacokinetics of high dose mebendazole in patients treated for cystic hydatid disease. European Journal of Clinical Pharmacology. 1982;**22**:161-169

[8] de Silva NR, Sirisena JL, Gunasekera DP, Ismail MM, de Silva HJ. Effect of mebendazole therapy during pregnancy on birth outcome. Lancet. 1999;**353**:1145-1149

[9] Velasco-Tirado V, Alonso-Sardón M, Lopez-Bernus A, Romero-Alegría Á, Burguillo FJ, Muro A, et al. Medical treatment of cystic echinococcosis: Systematic review and meta-analysis. BMC Infectious Diseases. 2018;**18**(1):306

[10] Dumitru IM, Dumitru E, Rugină S. Role of epidemiologic data in management of hydatidosis in Constanta County, Romania. Therapeutics Pharmacology and Clinical Toxicology. 2011;**15**(2):132-138

[11] Dumitru IM, Dumitru E, Rugină S, Dumitru A. The albendazole treatment's efficacy in hydatid cysts. Therapeutics Pharmacology and Clinical Toxicology. 2015;**19**(1):19-22

[12] Dumitru IM, Cernat RC, Dumitru E, Rugina S. Cystic Echinococcosis in HIV infected patients. The XXVIth World Congress on Echinococcosis. 2015;**43**(3):44-45

[13] Anand S, Rajagopalan S, Mohan R. Management of liver hydatid cysts—Current perspectives. Medical Journal, Armed Forces India. 2012;**68**(3):304-309

[14] Mortezaei S, Afgar A, Mohammadi MA, Mousavi SM, Sadeghi B, Harandi MF. The effect of albendazole sulfoxide on the expression of miR-61 and let-7 in different in vitro developmental stages of *Echinococcus granulosus*. Acta Tropica. 2019;**195**:97-102

[15] Hemphill A, Stadelmann B, Scholl S, Müller J, Spiliotis M, Müller N, et al. Echinococcus metacestodes as laboratory models for the screening of drugs against cestodes and trematodes. Parasitology. 2010;**137**:569-587

[16] Karabulut K, Ozbalci GS, Kesicioglu T, Tarim IA, Lap G, Kamali Polat A, et al. Long-term outcomes of intraoperative and perioperative albendazole treatment in hepatic hydatidosis: Single center experience. Annals of Surgical Treatment and Research. 2014;**87**:61-65

[17] Horton RJ. Chemotherapy of Echinococcus infection in man with albendazole. Transactions of the Royal Society of Tropical Medicine and Hygiene. 1989;**83**:97-102

[18] Loos JA, Cumino AC. In vitro anti-echinococcal and metabolic effects of metformin involve activation of AMP-activated protein kinase in larval stages of *Echinococcus granulosus*. PLoS One. 12 May 2015;**10**(5):e0126009

[19] Loos JA, Dávila VA, Rodrígues CR, Petrigh R, Zoppi JA, Crocenzi FA, et al. Metformin exhibits preventive and therapeutic efficacy against experimental cystic echinococcosis. PLoS Neglected Tropical Diseases. 2 Mar 2017;**11**(3):e0005474

[20] Gorgas D, Marreros N, Rufener R, Hemphill A, Lundström-Stadelmann B. To see or not to see: Non-invasive imaging for improved readout of drug treatment trials in the murine model of secondary alveolar echinococcosis. Parasitology. 2017;**144**(7):937-944

[21] Panwar P, Pandey B, Lakhera PC, Singh KP. Preparation, characterization, and in vitro release study of albendazole-encapsulated nanosize liposomes. International Journal of Nanomedicine. 2010;**5**:101-108

[22] Bygott JM, Chiodini PL. Praziquantel: Neglected drug? Ineffective treatment? Or therapeutic choice in cystic hydatid disease? Acta Tropica. 2009;**111**:95-101

[23] Jamshidi M, Mohraz M, Zangeneh M, Jamshidi A. The effect of combination therapy with albendazole and praziquantel on hydatid cyst treatment. Parasitology Research. 2008;**103**(1):195-199

[24] Jiang B, Zhou XN, Zhang HB, Tao Y, Huo LL, Liu N. Slow-release praziquantel for dogs: Presentation of a new formulation for echinococcosis control. Infectious Diseases of Poverty. 2017;**6**(1):140

[25] Cobo F, Yarnoz C, Sesma B, Fraile P, Aizcorbe M, Trujillo R, et al. Albendazole plus praziquantel versus albendazole alone as a pre-operative treatment in intra-abdominal hydatidosis caused by *Echinococcus granulosus*. Tropical Medicine and International Health. 1998;**3**(6):462-466

[26] Wen H, Vuitton L, Tuxun T, Li J, Vuitton DA, Zhang W, et al. Echinococcosis: Advances in the 21st century. Clinical Microbiology Reviews. 13 Feb 2019;**32**(2):pii: e00075-18.

[27] Hemphill A, Stadelmann B, Rufener R, Spiliotis M, Boubaker G, Müller J, et al. Treatment of echinococcosis: Albendazole and mebendazole—What else? Parasite. 2014;**21**:70

[28] Sanei B, Tavakoli P, Hadipour M, Darani HY. Effect of ursodeoxycholic acid, *Lawsonia inermis* and *Achillea millefolium* extracts on hydatid cyst protoscolices. Infectious Disorders Drug Targets. 5 Apr 2019. DOI: 10.2174/1871526519666190405142120. [Epub ahead of print]

[29] Xing G, Zhang H, Liu C, Guo Z, Yang X, Wang Z, et al. Sodium arsenite augments sensitivity of *Echinococcus granulosus* protoscoleces to albendazole. Experimental Parasitology. 2019;**200**:55-60

[30] Barzin Z, Sadjjadi SM, Panjehshahin MR. Protoscolicidal effects of the garlic chloroformic extract

on the protoscolices of hydatid cyst at a short exposure time, up to five minutes. Iranian Journal of Medical Sciences. 2019;**44**(1):28-34

[31] Rufener R, Dick L, D'Ascoli L, Ritler D, Hizem A, Wells TNC, et al. Repurposing of an old drug: In vitro and in vivo efficacies of buparvaquone against Echinococcus multilocularis. International Journal for Parasitology: Drugs and Drug Resistance. 2018;**8**(3):440-450

[32] Amiri K, Nasibi S, Mehrabani M, Nematollahi MH, Harandi MF. In vitro evaluation on the scolicidal effect of *Myrtus communis* L. and *Tripleurospermum disciforme* L. methanolic extracts. Experimental Parasitology. 2019;**199**:111-115

[33] Napooni S, Delavari M, Arbabi M, Barkheh H, Rasti S, Hooshyar H, et al. Scolicidal effects of chitosan-curcumin nanoparticles on the hydatid cyst protoscolices. Acta Parasitologica. Jun 2019;**64**(2):367-375

[34] Xu S, Duan L, Zhang H, Xu B, Chen J, Hu W, et al. In vitro efficacies of solubility-improved mebendazole derivatives against *Echinococcus multilocularis*. Parasitology. 6 May 2019: 1-7. DOI: 10.1017/S0031182019000386. [Epub ahead of print]

[35] Yuan M, Song X, Lv W, Xin Q, Wang L, Gao Q, et al. Effect of anacardic acid against echinococcosis through inhibition of VEGF-induced angiogenesis. Veterinary Research. 2019;**50**(1):3

[36] Kammerer WS, Perez-Esandi MV. Chemotherapy of experimental *Echinococcus granulosus* infection. Trials in CF1 mice and jirds (*Meriones unguiculatus*). The American Journal of Tropical Medicine and Hygiene. 1975;**24**(1):90-95

[37] Miyaji S, Katakura K, Matsufuji S, Murakami Y, Hayashi S, Oku Y, et al. Failure of treatment with alpha-difluoromethylornithine against secondary multilocular echinococcosis in mice. Parasitology Research. 1993;**79**(1):75-76

[38] Reuter S, Manfras B, Merkle M, Härter G, Kern P. In vitro activities of itraconazole, methiazole, and nitazoxanide versus Echinococcus multilocularis larvae. Antimicrobial Agents and Chemotherapy. 2006;**50**(9):2966-2970

[39] Reuter S, Beisler T, Kern P. Combined albendazole and amphotericin B against *Echinococcus multilocularis* in vitro. Acta Tropica. 2010;**115**(3):270-274

[40] Reuter S, Buck A, Grebe O, Nüssle-Kügele K, Kern P, Manfras BJ. Salvage treatment with amphotericin B in progressive human alveolar echinococcosis. Antimicrobial Agents and Chemotherapy. 2003;**47**(11):3586-3591

[41] Reuter S, Merkle M, Brehm K, Kern P, Manfras B. Effect of amphotericin B on larval growth of *Echinococcus multilocularis*. Antimicrobial Agents and Chemotherapy. 2003;**47**(2):620-625

[42] Tappe D, Müller A, Frosch M, Stich A. Limitations of amphotericin B and nitazoxanide in the treatment of alveolar echinococcosis. Annals of Tropical Medicine and Parasitology. 2009;**103**(2):177-181

[43] Stettler M, Rossignol JF, Fink R, Walker M, Gottstein B, Merli M, et al. Secondary and primary murine alveolar echinococcosis: Combined albendazole/nitazoxanide chemotherapy exhibits profound anti-parasitic activity. International Journal for Parasitology. 2004;**34**(5):615-624

[44] Stettler M, Fink R, Walker M, Gottstein B, Geary TG, Rossignol JF,

et al. In vitro parasiticidal effect of Nitazoxanide against Echinococcus multilocularis metacestodes. Antimicrobial Agents and Chemotherapy. 2003;**47**(2):467-474

[45] Walker M, Rossignol JF, Torgerson P, Hemphill A. In vitro effects of nitazoxanide on *Echinococcus granulosus* protoscoleces and metacestodes. The Journal of Antimicrobial Chemotherapy. 2004;**54**(3):609-616

[46] Winning A, Braslins P, McCarthy JS. Case report: Nitazoxanide for treatment of refractory bony hydatid disease. The American Journal of Tropical Medicine and Hygiene. 2009;**80**(2):176-178

[47] Bonilla M, Denicola A, Novoselov SV, Turanov AA, Protasio A, Izmendi D, et al. Platyhelminth mitochondrial and cytosolic redox homeostasis is controlled by a single thioredoxin glutathione reductase and dependent on selenium and glutathione. The Journal of Biological Chemistry. 2008;**283**(26):17898-17907

[48] Ross F, Hernández P, Porcal W, López GV, Cerecetto H, González M, et al. Identification of thioredoxin glutathione reductase inhibitors that kill cestode and trematode parasites. PLoS One. 2012;**7**(4):e35033

[49] Saiz C, Castillo V, Fontán P, Bonilla M, Salinas G, Rodríguez-Haralambides A, et al. Discovering *Echinococcus granulosus* thioredoxin glutathione reductase inhibitors through site-specific dynamic combinatorial chemistry. Molecular Diversity. 2014;**18**(1):1-12

[50] Salinas G, Gao W, Wang Y, Bonilla M, Yu L, Novikov A, et al. The enzymatic and structural basis for inhibition of *Echinococcus granulosus* thioredoxin glutathione reductase by gold (I). Antioxidants & Redox Signaling. 2017;**27**(18):1491-1504

[51] Stadelmann B, Küster T, Scholl S, Barna F, Kropf C, Keiser J, et al. In vitro efficacy of dicationic compounds and mefloquine enantiomers against *Echinococcus multilocularis* metacestodes. Antimicrobial Agents and Chemotherapy. 2011;**55**(10):4866-4872

[52] Küster T, Stadelmann B, Hermann C, Scholl S, Keiser J, Hemphill A. In vitro and in vivo efficacies of mefloquine-based treatment against alveolar echinococcosis. Antimicrobial Agents and Chemotherapy. 2011;**55**(2):713-721

[53] Küster T, Stadelmann B, Rufener R, Risch C, Müller J, Hemphill A. Oral treatments of *Echinococcus multilocularis*-infected mice with the antimalarial drug mefloquine that potentially interacts with parasite ferritin and cystatin. International Journal of Antimicrobial Agents. 2015;**46**(5):546-551

[54] Rufener R, Ritler D, Zielinski J, Dick L, da Silva ET, da Silva Araujo A, et al. Activity of mefloquine and mefloquine derivatives against *Echinococcus multilocularis*. International Journal for Parasitology: Drugs and Drug Resistance. 2018;**8**(2):331-340

[55] Labsi M, Soufli I, Khelifi L, Amir ZC, Touil-Boukoffa C. A preventive effect of the combination of albendazole and pomegranate peel aqueous extract treatment in cystic Echinococcosis mice model: An alternative approach. Acta Tropica. 2019;**197**:105050. DOI: 10.1016/j.actatropica.2019.105050. [Epub ahead of print]

[56] Tabari MA, Youssefi MR, Nasiri M, Hamidi M, Kiani K, Alian Samakkhah S, et al. Towards green drugs against cestodes: Effectiveness of *Pelargonium roseum* and *Ferula gummosa* essential oils and their main

component on *Echinococcus granulosus* protoscoleces. Veterinary Parasitology. 2019;**266**:84-87

[57] Siles-Lucas M, Casulli A, Cirilli R, Carmena D. Progress in the pharmacological treatment of human cystic and alveolar echinococcosis: Compounds and therapeutic targets. PLoS Neglected Tropical Diseases. 2018;**12**(4):e0006422

[58] Ochieng'-Mitula PJ, Burt MD. The effects of ivermectin on the hydatid cyst of *Echinococcus granulosus* after direct injection at laparotomy. The Journal of Parasitology. 1996;**82**:155-157

[59] Hurd H, Mackenzie KS, Chappell LH. Anthelmintic effects of cyclosporin A on protoscoleces and secondary hydatid cysts of *Echinococcus granulosus* in the mouse. International Journal for Parasitology. 1993;**23**:315-320

[60] Schubert A, Koziol U, Cailliau K, Vanderstraete M, Dissous C, Brehm K. Targeting *Echinococcus multilocularis* stem cells by inhibition of the Polo-like kinase EmPlk1. PLoS Neglected Tropical Diseases. 2014;**8**:e2870

[61] Ullio Gamboa GV, Pensel PE, Elissondo MC, Sanchez Bruni SF, Benoit JP, Palma SD, et al. Albendazole-lipid nanocapsules: Optimization, characterization and chemoprophylactic efficacy in mice infected with *Echinococcus granulosus*. Experimental Parasitology. 2019;**198**:79-86

[62] Zhao X, Zhang F, Li Z, Wang H, An M, Li Y, et al. Bioinformatics analysis of EgA31 and EgG1Y162 proteins for designing a multi-epitope vaccine against *Echinococcus granulosus*. Infection, Genetics and Evolution. 2019;**73**:98-108

[63] Miles S, Portela M, Cyrklaff M, Ancarola ME, Frischknecht F, Durán R, et al. Combining proteomics and bioinformatics to explore novel tegumental antigens as vaccine candidates against *Echinococcus granulosus* infection. Journal of Cellular Biochemistry. Sep 2019;**120**(9):15320-15336

[64] Larrieu E, Mujica G, Araya D, Labanchi JL, Arezo M, Herrero E, et al. Pilot field trial of the EG95 vaccine against ovine cystic echinococcosis in Rio Negro, Argentina: 8 years of work. Acta Tropica. 2019;**191**:1-7

[65] Liu F, Fan X, Li L, Ren W, Han X, Wu X, et al. Development of recombinant goatpox virus expressing *Echinococcus granulosus* EG95 vaccine antigen. Journal of Virological Methods. 2018;**261**:28-33

[66] Liu F, Li L, Liu Y, Sun C, Liu C, Wu X, et al. Development of reverse genetics system for small ruminant morbillivirus: Rescuing recombinant virus to express *Echinococcus granulosus* EG95 antigen. Virus Research. 2019;**261**:50-55

Chapter 7

Utility of ERCP in the Diagnosis and Management of Biliary Complications of Hepatic Hydatid Disease

Pedro Pinto, Sergio Gaete and Patricia Vega

Abstract

To report the experience with endoscopic retrograde cholangiopancreatography (ERCP) in the pre- and postoperative management of complicated liver hydatidosis. Case series retrospective of 14 patients who underwent ERCP in the Department of Surgery and Endoscopy Regional Hospital of Coyhaique, from January 2005 to December 2014. In this report, patients are separated into two groups: those in whom ERCP was used as diagnosis and those in which it was used for handling the external biliary fistula. Five patients consulting for jaundice and pain were subjected to ERCP in the preoperative period. Hydatid membranes were found and extracted in all. A sphincterotomy was performed in all, and an endoprosthesis was placed in one. Four patients were operated posteriorly, and only one did not require surgery. On nine patients with an external biliary fistula draining more than 200 ml/day, a postoperative ERCP was carried out. The surgical procedure was a partial cystectomy, and in four it was laparoscopic. The ERCP was carried out in the 20th postoperative day, performing a sphincterotomy and placing an endoprosthesis in all. Fistulae are closed at 28 days. Patients were followed up for 6 years and none died.

Keywords: hepatic hydatid cyst, complications, biliary fistula, endoscopic pancreatography

1. Introduction

The liver is compromised in 50–70% of patients with hydatid disease. The most frequent hepatic hydatid cyst (HCH) complication is intrabiliary rupture, which occurs in 5–25% of patients. This rupture can lead to the obstruction of the Bile duct cholangitis and sepsis which can reach 50% of mortality. Surgery has been the traditional treatment for these patients, which has been associated with a high morbidity ranging 21.3–53.8% according to several series [1], the external biliary fistula (EBF) being the most frequent complication with 4–28% of the total [2].

Since the first communication in 1987 about the endoscopic retrograde cholangiopancreatography (ERPC) utility in the study and treatment of patients with complicated hepatic hydatidosis (CHH) [3, 4], more than 1000 patients had undergone this procedure, with a complication rate of 7.9% and a mortality of 0.6% [5].

The ERPC is mainly used in the preoperative period to solve acute complications such as cholangitis and the obstruction of the bile duct cystic material and in the postoperative management of the EBF and benign strictures of the biliary duct [6].

The aim of this presentation is to report the surgery and endoscopy service experience in the use of ERPC, in both pre- and postoperative stages of CHH patients.

2. Material and method

Retrospective case series from 14 patients are submitted to ERPC in the Department of Surgery and Endoscopy Regional Hospital of Coyhaique, from January 2005 to December 2014. Such procedure was used in the pre- and postoperative handling of patients with CHH.

During this period, 218 CHH carrying patients were treated, and 9 (4.1%) of them presented EBF high drainage complications; therefore they will be the reason for this presentation. In turn, the endoscopy service realized 832 ERPC during the same period, and only 14 (1.7%) presented CHH as an indication.

In this presentation, patients are separated into two groups: those in whom ERCP was used as diagnosis (**Table 1**) and those in which it was used for managing the external biliary fistula (**Table 2**).

In a previous post [7], it is established that biliary fistula refers to a bile flow which extends for more than 10 days. The draining qualifies as low when the flow is less than 200 ml per day and high when it is greater than that quantity. The ERPC indication was an average biliary draining greater than 200 cc per day.

The ERPC was performed by the endoscopy unit team at the Imaging Service of the Coyhaique Regional Hospital. All patients underwent antibioprophylaxis with 1 g of intravenous cefazolin, they were sedated with midazolam and fentanyl, and the peristalsis duodenal was suppressed with hyoscine butylbromide

Patient no.	Age	Sex	Clinic	Ultrasound	ERPC findings	ERPC technique	Monitoring
1	76	F	Jaundice	SVI-SVII, MV, 12 × 7 cm, communicated to BD	Cholangiohydatidosis	Membrane extraction sphincterotomy	Operated the following month
2	55	M	Jaundice	SV-SVI, UV, 11 × 6 cm	Communication BD cyst	Sphincterotomy	Operated 2 months later
3	51	M	Jaundice	Caudate lobe, MV 48 × 37 × 47 mm	Cholangiohydatidosis	Membrane extraction sphincterotomy	Not operated Medical examinations ok
4	35	M	Jaundice, pain	SII-SIII, MV, 13 cm	Cholangiohydatidosis	Membrane extraction sphincterotomy endoprosthesis 7.5 F	Operated the following month
5	55	M	Jaundice, pain	RHL, 17 × 13 × 13 cm communicated to BD, hepatic hilum	Cholangiohydatidosis communication right hepatic	Membrane extraction sphincterotomy	Operated 20 days later

Table 1.
Diagnosis.

Patient no.	Age	Sex	Hepatic hydatid cyst (intraoperative) location-size-characteristic	Surgical technique	Lapse ERPC/surgery days (bile flow)	ERPC technique	Monitoring
1	49	M	SIV: 6 x 5 cm, MV bilis 5 x 4 cm, MV	Indirect marsupialization	13 days (300 ml)	Endoprosthesis 7 F papillotomy	30/50
2	63	M	SVII-SVIII, 11 × 11 × 10 cm, MV bilis output can be seen	LC partial cystectomy	15 days (250 ml)	Endoprosthesis 7 F papillotomy (2 ERPC)	11/48
3	33	F	SII-III, 15 × 20 cm bilobulated	LC partial cystectomy LC	27 days (400 ml)	2 endoprosthesis 7 F	14/39
4	70	M	3: SV, 19 × 17cm, UV SVIII, 15 × 13 cm, MV bilis SII, 8 × 9 cm, MV bilis	Partial cystectomy capitonnage partial resection	10 days (250 ml)	Endoprosthesis 8.5 F papillotomy	34/42
5	11	M	SVIII (2), 10 and 4 cm, MV	Partial cystectomy	25 days (800 ml)	Endoprosthesis 7 F papillotomy	9/126
6	45	M	SII-SIII, 15 × 13 cm, UV frank bilis	Partial cystectomy	11 days (1000 ml)	Endoprosthesis 7 F papillotomy	37/129
7	54	M	Between LHL and RHL, 12 × 10 × 11 cm, UV, frank bilis	LC	7 days (200 ml)	Endoprosthesis 7 F papillotomy	31/71
8	10	M	LHL, 10 × 12 cm, MV, ruptured peritoneum	Partial cystectomy	41 days (300 ml)	Endoprosthesis 7 F, 2 ERPC performed	57/120
9	13	M	RHL 17 × 9.5 × 11.8 cm, UV, bilis	Partial cystectomy	27 days (990 ml)	Endoprosthesis 8.5 F papillotomy	28/18

ERPC, endoscopic pancreatography; F, frank; F, female ("sex" column); RHL, right hepatic lobe; LHL, left hepatic lobe; M, male; MV, multivesicular; LC, laparoscopic cystectomy; S, segment; UV, univesicular.

Table 2.
External bilary fistula management.

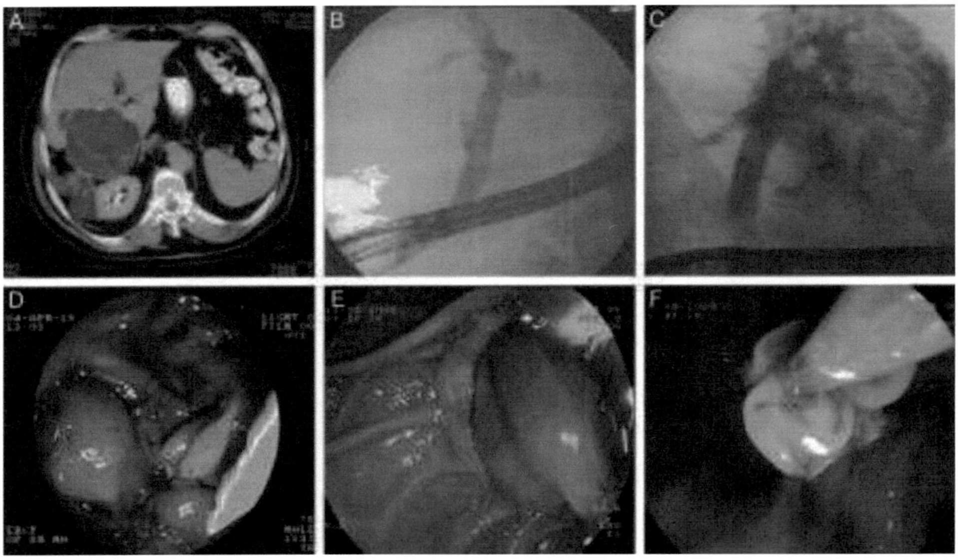

Figure 1.
(A) HHC CAT image. (B) Hydatid material in the common biliary duct. (C) Extravasation of contrast media from the biliary ducts to the cystic cavity. (D) Hydatid material infected post-papillotomy draining. (E) Hydatid material extraction through an endoscopic balloon. (F) Way out of germinative from the choledochal.

of scopolamine. The procedure was performed with the patient in the left lateral decubitus position using the EXERA TJF-160VF OLYMPUS videodenoscope. The sphincterotomy was performed in the classic way with a TRI-20M papillotome (TR-TOME PC triple lumen COOK) guided with HYB-48015. After the sphincterotomy was done, a Dormia MSN COOK canister or a TXR COOK balloon was used to extract the daughter vesicles and to allow a fluid biliary drainage.

ERPC, endoscopic pancreatography; F, frank; F, female ("sex" column); RHL, right hepatic lobe; M, male; MV, multivesicular; S, segment; BD, biliary duct.

If stenting was required, an Oasis set of prosthesis introduction (OACL, 7.5–10 F) was used (**Figure 1**).

After discharge, patients were followed a month later, 3 and 6 months later, and then 1 year later.

3. Results

There were five patients submitted to ERPC in the preoperative period (**Table 1**). Male sex predominated and the average age was 54 ± 15 years old. The average cyst size was 12 ± 4.4 cm and all of them were multivesicular.

The main consultation motive was jaundice and pain, only one of them had as an antecedent having undergone a CHH surgery. In all of them, a passage of hydatid membranes to the main bile duct was found and endoscopically extracted. Sphincterotomy was performed in all, and only one case required an endoprosthesis installation which was subsequently removed (**Figure 1**).

Four patients were stabilized and operated according to schedule before a month, and only the one who had the minor-sized cyst (48 × 37 × 47 mm) located in the caudate lobe did not require surgery, and his examinations are normal until now.

Due to the EBF presence with sustained high output (>200 ml) bile flow, ERPC was performed in nine patients aiming to close it (**Table 2**). As in the preoperative therapeutic use, male sex predominates, and the average age was 39 ± 22 years. The cyst size was 12 ± 5 cm, and two thirds of them were multivesicular.

The surgical technique employed in all was non-resective (partial cystectomy), and in four patients (4/9) it was performed through a videolaparoscopy. ERPC indication took place 20 days (7–41) after the intervention, and the average EBF output was 498 ml per day (200–1000). Sphincterotomy was performed in all with endoprosthesis installation, mostly 7F (7/9). The fistula closure happened on average at 28 ± 15 days. The prosthesis was extracted from five patients between week 6 and 8 after the EBF.

The patients' monitoring reached 71.4 ± 42 months (6 years), with a minimum of 18 and a maximum of 129 months (10.7 years).

4. Discussion

So far we have only found one work in literature published by national authors related to the utility of ERPC in CHH [8] and hence the interest in making it known.

The communication among CHH and the biliary tree is the most frequent and severe complication, and it explains 60% of the complications. When this communication is greater than 5 mm, it is called frank rupture, and in 65% of the cases, it is possible to see cystic content in the main biliary duct [9]. The classic treatment for these patients was surgery; however, since Al Karawi et al. in 1987 [3] reported the use of ERPC with sphincterotomy in the handling of daughter vesicles retained in the biliary duct, this procedure has been considered as a safe and effective choice.

ERPC is used in the preoperative period with the following objectives [10]:

- Surgery planning by defining the cystobiliar relationship.
- Resolution of acute conditions such as cholangitis and obstruction of the main bile duct, allowing elective surgery (cases 1, 2, 4, and 5).
- In 25% of cases, it allows for a permanent cure [3, 11], which is confirmed in our series (case 3).
- Complementing the procedure with sphincterotomy reduces the incidence of EBF.

In the postoperative period, its main indications are [10]:

- Solving the obstruction and the cholangitis caused by the presence of hydatid material in the bile ducts.
- Enabling the best handling of EBF (1–9 cases).
- Solving the secondary biliary stenosis to the CHH.

It is essential to bear in mind that the ERPC indication must be precocious, ideally within 10 days after the EBF has been established [12].

The main problem is in low output fistula. According to Zeybek et al. when the flow is 102 ml per day, this closes spontaneously [13], and the end of the flow occurs 34.7 days [7] later; therefore, there is a tendency to have an expectant behavior due to the inherent risks of the procedure.

The fistula high output case is different, in which aggressive behavior is required, since the stay of these patients is even longer (41.6 days) [7] and the risk of complications increases. The average output in our patients reached 498 ml per day, and the ERPC indication was performed when the flow was persistently greater than 200 mh and the latency of the procedure reached 20 days, a situation that we have tried to correct in the last patients.

When reviewing the worldwide experience up to 2002 in the endoscopic management of CHH, the Turkish gastroenterologists Ersan Özaslan and Yusuf Bayraktar mention that optimal management of EBF remains unanswered. In their opinion of sphincterotomy, stent and nasobiliar drainage are not exclusive but complementary, and each should be used according to the individual characteristic of each patient [6].

The therapy performed in the service to patients with EBF consisted of a combination of sphincterotomy plus stent installation. In the first patients a 7 F was used to subsequently use a thicker 8.5 F. This was done to reduce the probability of being obstructed with the content of the residual cavity and having to change and reinstall it, as occurred in two patients.

All this was subsequently endorsed by the publication of Adas et al. [14], who in a retrospective multicenter study concluded that sphincterotomy is the treatment of choice in low debit EBFs, but in high debit EBFs (flow greater than 200 ml per day), the gold standard is the insertion of a 10 F stent whenever possible.

It is worth mentioning that the removal of the prosthesis should not be performed beyond 4–6 weeks after the cessation of EBF [12]. In our patients this was performed in 5 of 9, those in which choledocholithiasis was not favored, thus requiring a new ERCP (patient 7), in another there was persistence of infection of the residual cavity (patient 2), in a third the stent had to be removed due to persistent pain (patient 3), and in another there was migration of the prosthesis to the residual cavity (patient 9). Therefore, at this time, as a rule, the stent is removed no later than 4–6 weeks after the cessation of bile flow.

According to the different series, the objective of the cessation of EBF is achieved by 83.3–100%, and the closing time varies between 2 and 4 weeks [12]. When reviewing our series, the target was 100%, and the average closing time of the EBF was 28 days. This is far from the spontaneous evolution that reached 42 days in a previous publication [7].

It is worth mentioning that the monitoring of patients in this series of cases reached 100%, the average being 6 years. This occurs because the disease mainly affects patients who are beneficiaries of the public system, and since there is no private clinic in the region, in most cases they must be controlled in the regional hospital.

In this series of cases, there was no mortality.

5. Conclusions

This study confirms that ERPC is a useful and safe procedure in the diagnosis and treatment of bile complications of liver hydatidosis.

Conflict of interest

The authors declare no conflict of interest.

Notes/thanks/other declarations

None.

Author details

Pedro Pinto[1*], Sergio Gaete[2] and Patricia Vega[2]

1 Surgery Service, Coyhaique Regional Hospital, Coyhaique, Chile

2 Endoscopy Unit, Coyhaique Regional Hospital, Coyhaique, Chile

*Address all correspondence to: pedropablopatricio@gmail.com

References

[1] Manterola C, Urrutia S. Morbilidad postoperatoria en pacientes con hidatidosis hepática complicada. Revista Chilena de Infectología. 2015;**32**(1):43-49

[2] Singh V, Reddy DC, Verma GR, Singh G. Endoscopic management of intrabiliary-ruptured hepatic hydatid cyst. Liver International. 2006;**26**(5):621-624

[3] Al Karawi MA, Mohamed AE, Yasawy I, Haleem A. Non-surgical endoscopic trans-papillary treatment of ruptured echinococcosis liver cyst obstructing the biliary tree. Endoscopy. 1987;**19**(2):81-83

[4] Al Karawi MA, Yazawy MI, El Sheikh FS, Mohamed AR. Endoscopic management of biliary hydatid disease. Report on six cases. Endoscopy. 1991;**23**(5):278-281

[5] Rabenstein T, Schneider HT, Hahn EG, Ell C. 25 years of endoscopic sphincterotomy in Erlangen: Assessment of the experience in 3.498 patients. Endoscopy. 1998;**30**(2):194-201

[6] Ozaslan E, Bayraktar Y. Endoscopic therapy in the management of hepatobiliary hydatid disease. Journal of Clinical Gastroenterology. 2002;**35**(2):160-174

[7] Pinto P, López R. Evolución natural de la fístula biliar externa post cirugía del quiste hidatídico hepático. Revista Chilena de Cirugía. 2010;**62**(5):476-479

[8] De Aretxabala X, Pérez OL. The use of endoprótesis in biliary fistula of hydatid cyst. Gastrointestinal Endoscopy. 1999;**49**(6):797-799

[9] Zaouche A, Haouet K, Jovini M, El Hachaichi A, Dziri C. Management of liver hydatid cyst with a large biliocystic fistula: Multicenter retrospective study. World Journal of Surgery. 2001;**25**(1):28-39

[10] Ozaslan E. Therapeutic endoscopic retrograde cholangiopancreatography and related modalities have many roles in hepatobiliary hydatid disease. World Journal of Gastroenterology. 2006;**12**(30):4930-4931

[11] Dolay K, Akbulut S. Role of endoscopic retrograde cholangiopancreatography in the management of hepatic hydatid disease. World Journal of Gastroenterology. 2014;**20**(41):15253-15261

[12] Akcakaya A, Sahin M, Karakelleoglu A, Okan I. Endoscopic stenting for selected cases of biliary fistula after hepatic hydatid surgery. Surgical Endoscopy. 2006;**20**(9):1415-1418

[13] Zeybek N, Dede H, Balci D, Coskun AK, Ozerhan IH, Peker S, et al. Biliary fistula after treatment for hydatid disease of the liver: When to intervene. World Journal of Gastroenterology. 2013;**19**(3):355-361

[14] Adas G, Arikan S, Gurbuz E, Karahan S, Eryasar B, Karatepe O, et al. Comparison of endoscopic therapeutic modalities for postoperative biliary fistula of liver hydatid cyst: A retrospective multicentric study. Surgical Laparoscopy, Endoscopy & Percutaneous Techniques. 2010;**20**(49):223-227

Chapter 8

The Surgical Management of Hydatid Cyst of the Liver: What is New?

Mehmet Mihmanli, Mert Tanal, Emre Bozkurt and Onur Guven

Abstract

Liver hydatid cyst is a disease of zoonosis caused by *Echinococcus granulosus* or less frequently by *Echinococcus multilocularis* and *Echinococcus oligarthrus*. The primary carriers are canines, while human beings are secondary hosts. Early diagnosis is important for cysts not to become complicated and for the treatment not to get difficult. The most effective treatment of uncomplicated hydatid cyst is to reduce the dead space of the cavity and to discharge the fluid as much as possible. However, if the cysts get complex, there is no standard treatment management defined other than offered management options by authors. In complex conditions, the treatment is determined according to the stage of the cyst and the relation of the cyst with biliary ducts or surrounding organs. In this chapter, the treatment regimens of liver hydatid disease mainly based on interventions and surgical operations are going to take a part.

Keywords: conservative surgery, *Echinococcus*, hydatid cyst, PAIR, radical surgery, zoonosis

1. Introduction

There are mainly three types of *Echinococcus* causing diseases in humans: *E. granulosus*, *E. alveolaris* (*E. multilocularis*), and *E. oligarthrus*. This chapter will be based on the surgical approaches to hydatid cysts caused by *E. granulosus*.

2. Pathophysiology

The agent of hydatid cysts is *Echinococcus granulosus* which belongs to the tapeworm family of cestodes. The tapeworm consists of four segments. The most important segment is the first segment, which consists of four hooked structures that help the pathogen attach to the tissues. The life cycle of the pathogen is unique and explains the pathology.

The hydatid cyst lesion has a round cystic structure and consists of three main layers: an external fibrous pericyst 2–4 mm thick, mainly composed of the host's tissues to protect itself from the cyst; 2-mm-thick middle, nucleus-free hyaline layer, also known as ectocyst, or the laminar membrane in other words; and parasitic inner germinal membrane, known as endocyst. The annual growth rate of the cysts is 1–3 cm per year.

The germinative layer on the wall of the cyst is the site of asexual proliferation and secretes the cystic fluid. The larvae also emerge from this layer. If the connections between the laminar layer and the pericyst layer break down, the oxygenation of the cyst deteriorates and cannot produce liquid. The inevitable consequence of this is that the growth of the cyst stops.

2.1 Life cycle of *E. granulosus*

The disease lives in canines that are infected by eating the internal organs of sheep which contain hydatid cysts. The eggs in the cysts adhere to the small intestines of the dogs and become adult tapeworms attached to the intestinal wall. Each worm holds about 500 ovaries in the intestine. Dog feces containing infected eggs contaminate grasses and farmland, and the ovaries are swallowed by intermediate hosts such as sheep, cattle, pigs, and humans. The egg has chitinous envelopes that are dissolved with gastric juice. The released ovary then passes through the intestinal mucosa and is transported by the portal vein to the liver, where it develops in an adult cyst. Most cysts are caught in hepatic sinusoids, and therefore 70% of hydatid cysts occur in the liver, often in the right inferior segments. The placed embryo is immediately transformed into larvae. The larvae turn to the vesicle (scolex) and to the cyst at the end. The larvae can multiply asexually. Thus, there may be more than one living larva in a single cyst. Several pathogens pass through the liver, and the lung keeps them in its capillary bed, or they enter to the systemic circulation to form cysts in the lungs, spleen, brain, or bones.

3. Diagnosis

Uncomplicated cysts may be silent and incidental. Rarely, the affected patient has symptoms such as right upper quadrant pain or abdominal distension. The cysts may be secondary infected (usually by *E. coli*), invade other organs, or even cause ruptures leading to an allergic or anaphylactic reaction.

There are four medical tests used in diagnosis: Casoni skin test, the complement fixation test, *Echinococcus* IHA (indirect hemagglutination) test, and enzyme-linked immunosorbent assay (ELISA). The Casoni skin test is no longer used. The complement fixation test (Weinberg) is not widely used in diagnosis (the sensitivity is about 80%), but it is useful in follow-up because it becomes negative after the first year of the treatment. Its sensitivity is about 90% by then.

The *Echinococcus* IHA (indirect hemagglutination) is the most commonly used diagnostic test in practice. Its sensitivity is 90%. The *Echinococcus* IHA test is done by the patient's serum taken and diluted on microplates in times of 2, 4, 8, 16, 32, 64, 128, 256 ... 2048. A kit recognizing echinococcal antibodies is added to each microplate medium. If erythrocytes form agglutination in the presence of a kit, this indicates that the test is positive at that density. It is significant that IHA is positive at dilutions exceeding 1/128. However, many authors accept a 1/256 dilution as the presence of the disease. Positivity at lower dilutions means that the patient got cured or the disease is currently inactive.

It should be kept in mind that once IHA is positive, it may remain positive for more than 20 years. In a comprehensive epidemiological study published in Turkey, the positive prevalence of the *Echinococcus* IHA is 291/100,000 in the general population.

The diagnosis of hydatid cyst disease is based on the findings of ELISA for echinococcal antigens, and results are positive in approximately 85% of infected patients. The test may be negative if it is not leaking or the parasite is no longer alive.

In conclusion, the serological screening tests based on antigens (e.g., indirect hemagglutination, latex agglutination, ELISA) are highly associated with false-positive and false-negative results. However, while ELISA detection of specific antigens and immune complexes of the cyst has a much higher sensitivity, ELISA and radioallergosorbent test (RAST) can also detect specific IgE antibodies. Antigen 5 (arc-5) and antigen B8 are the major parasitic antigens having diagnostic value.

Eosinophilia occurs in approximately 30% of infected patients. Ultrasonography and CT scan of the abdomen are very sensitive in hydatid cyst detection, and the appearance of cysts on images depends on the stage of cyst development. Ultrasound images may show peripheral calcifications of cysts or curved bands of delaminated endocysts, called lotus. In CT scans, hydatid cysts are usually seen as hypodense lesions.

Calcification of female cysts occurs in approximately 75% of cases and 50% of the surrounding cyst wall [1]. As healing occurs, the entire cyst densely calcifies, and a lesion with this appearance is usually dead or ineffective. Daughter cysts usually occur at a peripheral location within the mother cyst and are typically more hypodense than the mother cyst. Abdominal MRI may be useful in assessing pericyst, cyst matrix, and daughter cyst characteristics. MRI is the technique that best shows pericyst or "cyst hydatid sand" (free floating membranes) and daughter cysts. Fibrous and rigid pericysts appear as a hypodense ring on both T1- and T2-weighted images. The hydatid matrix is hyperdense in T2-weighted images and hypodense in T1-weighted images. Daughter cysts may be seen in both T1- and T2-weighted images.

The treatment and the follow-up procedures are based on the cyst and the symptoms of the patients. Below, you may find the clinical and radiological staging as well as WHO classification for hydatid cysts.

3.1 Clinical staging

Stage 1: Asymptomatic.

Stage 2: Symptomatic (right upper quadrant pain).

Stage 3: Symptomatic + presence of liver dysfunction (e.g., AST, ALT elevation).

3.2 Gharbi classification in USG

Type 1: Pure liquid collection.

Type 2: The decomposition of the germinative membrane and the pericyst.

Type 3: Multivesicular type.

Type 4: Heterogeneous echo pattern.

Type 5: The calcified wall.

3.3 2001 WHO classification

- CL
    - Unilocular anechoic cystic lesion [2]
    - No any internal echoes or septations

- **CE 1** (active stage)
  - Uniformly anechoic cyst with fine internal echoes, may only be visible after patient repositioning (**Figure 1**).
  - Internal echoes represent "hydatid sand" (fluid and protoscolices originating from a ruptured vesicle).
- **CE 2** (active stage)
  - Cyst with internal septation (**Figure 2**)
  - Septa represent walls of daughter cyst(s)
  - Described as multivesicular, rosette, or honeycomb appearance
- **CE 3** (transitional stage)
  - Evolving appearance of daughter cyst(s) within the encompassing parent cyst
  - **3A**—daughter cysts have detached laminated membranes (water lily sign) (**Figure 3**)
  - **3B**—daughter cysts within a solid matrix

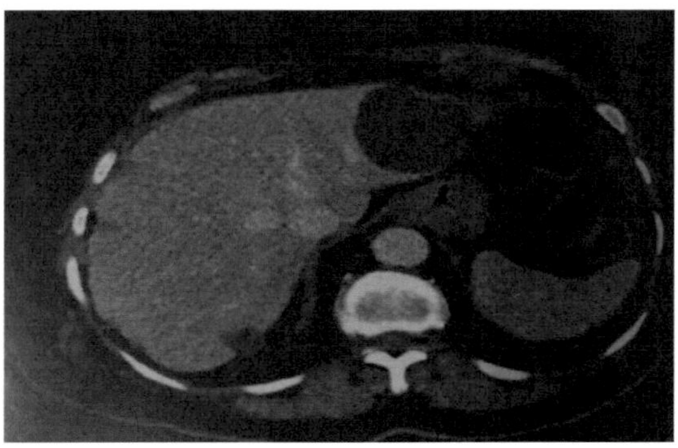

Figure 1.
CE1 hydatid cyst in both liver lobes shown in abdominal CT scan [3].

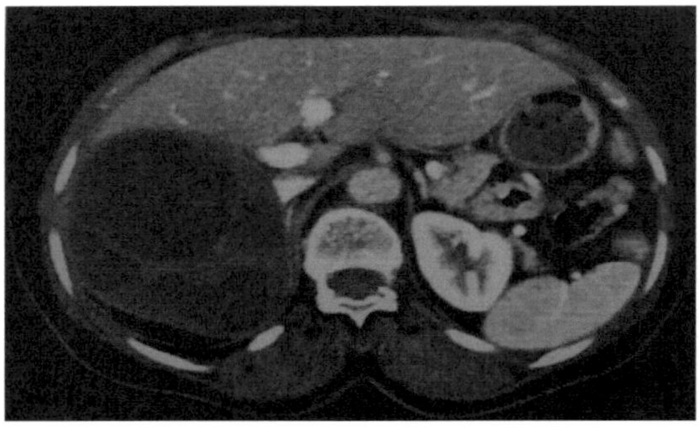

Figure 2.
CE2 hydatid cyst in right liver lobe shown in abdominal CT scan [3].

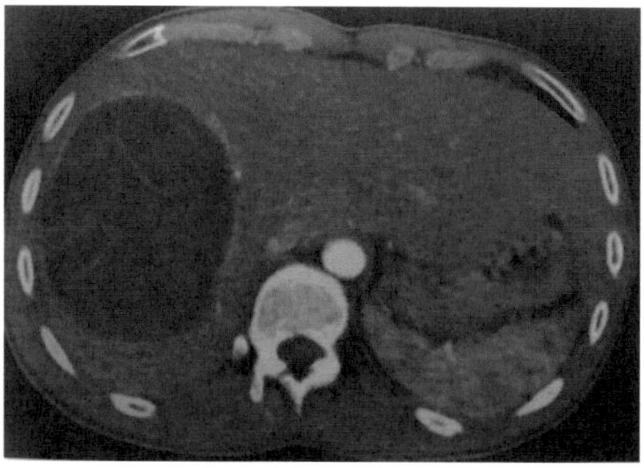

Figure 3.
CE3a hydatid cyst in right liver lobe shown in abdominal CT scan [3].

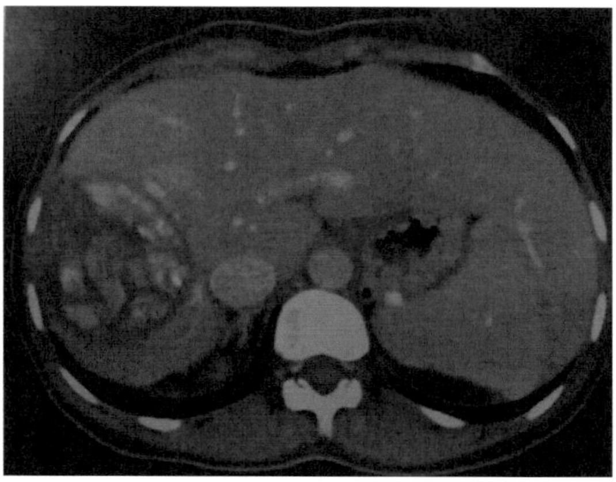

Figure 4.
CE4 hydatid cyst in right liver lobe shown in abdominal CT scan [3].

- **CE 4** (inactive/degenerative)
    - Absence of daughter cysts (**Figure 4**)
    - Mixed hypoechoic and hyperechoic matrix, resembling a ball of wool (ball of wool sign)
- **CE 5** (inactive/degenerative)
    - Arch-like, thick partially or completely calcified wall

4. The medical treatment

The goal of the treatment is mainly to stop the growth of the cyst and to eliminate the risk of infection or rupture. Unless the cysts are small, cyst hydatid disease is treated surgically because of high risk of secondary infection and rupture. Benzimidazole-derived antibiotics such as mebendazole and its new analogue albendazole are used. Medical treatment with albendazole relies on drug diffusion along the cyst membrane. The concentration of drug obtained in the cyst is uncertain but is better than that of mebendazole, and albendazole can be used as an initial treatment for small, asymptomatic cysts.

The standard dose of mebendazole is 35–50 mg/kg/day, and the standard administration period is 6 months, whereas albendazole's standard dose is 10 mg/kg/day. Albendazole is more effective than mebendazole, because it has better absorption from the gastrointestinal tract, reaching much higher concentrations in both serum and cyst fluids. Therefore, the daily dose of albendazole is lower. However, it has toxic effects on the liver and bone marrow. For this reason, liver function tests and hemogram should be performed periodically in the patients under treatment.

Even if the management of the patient is decided as operation, the administration of albendazole for 1 month preoperatively reduces the number of viable vesicles within the cyst and reduces the risk of surgical scattering/recurrence.

5. Interventional treatment algorithm

In the majority of the patients, the medical treatment of the hydatid cyst is applied first, both for the treatment of the disease and for reducing the rate of the complications even if the cure is going to be reached by the surgical procedures.

The effectivity of the medical treatment can be assessed in two ways. By radiological assessment, USG can be performed, and if the cyst diameter does not increase and/or calcification is developed, the medical treatment is successful. By the serological assessment, the IHA test is repeated after 6 months of treatment.

Regardless of the stage, special attention should be paid to the content of each cyst. Cysts, in which the content is biliary or purulent, deserve additional interventions (finding and suturing the biliary tract (s) opened to the cyst, making drainage more diligently, increasing the number of drains, etc.).

Even if the risk is first defined as 25% in literature [4], 5% of the cases with indication for surgery are associated with bile ducts. This risk is greater in multivesicular cysts. Biliary entrances may result from communication between the pericyst and the biliary tract or from rupture of the cyst into the biliary tract. Strong communication of the cysts and bile ducts can lead to secondary bacterial infection of the cyst, cholangitis, or biliary obstruction. Bacterial contamination occurs in 10–35% of cases, and almost all of the infected cysts are associated with bile ducts.

Occasionally, the cysts spontaneously tear into the peritoneal cavity and cause anaphylaxis, which starts with abdominal pain. Many intra-abdominal cysts may develop as a result of intraperitoneal leakage. Liver hydatid cysts can penetrate the diaphragm and cause empyema, pulmonary cysts, biliary bronchial fistulas, or pericardial collections.

Some hydatid cyst disintegrates into bile ducts and may simulate choledocholithiasis. If the calcified cyst is unclear, cholangiography may show significant irregularities in the caliber of biliary ducts and large displacement of intrahepatic branches secondary to the mass effect of a large hydatid cyst [5, 6]. Before the interventions, if the patient has signs of jaundice and/or cholangitis, preoperative MRCP and ERCP, if necessary, should be definitely evaluated for the presence of the cyst opening to the biliary tract or the presence of cysts in the biliary tract. This procedure is very important in determining the surgical strategy.

The general rule is that surgical treatment is indicated for cysts larger than 5 cm. However, there are controversial issues such as attempting medical treatment first or applying medical treatment if there already occurred calcification on the wall. The discussion remains under the knowledge of the physiology of the cyst.

6. Percutaneous techniques

Traditionally, surgery has been the recommended treatment for hepatic cysts since the 1996 World Health Organization Consortium [7], but the combination of percutaneous drainage with drug therapy is always an alternative. Although percutaneous aspiration is contraindicated due to the risk of anaphylaxis, this complication has been shown to be rare for many years [8, 9]. Initially, a catheter was inserted for percutaneous drainage, and a cystolytic agent was injected into the cyst cavity after cystography. No complications or recurrences were reported 6 months to 1 year after treatment.

If percutaneous drainage is planned for the patient, it is important to remember that hydatid cysts do not resolve by aspiration just like any cyst. Recurrence is almost inevitable when only aspiration is performed. Therefore, a percutaneous technique called PAIR (perforation, aspiration, injection, reaspiration) can be used concurrently with albendazole treatment, which is found to have several advantages over surgical resection. In this method, after ultrasound-guided percutaneous perforation and aspiration of the hydatid cyst, 20% sodium chloride solution or 95% ethanol is injected into the cavity and then reaspired [10]. This intervention can be done twice or more in the same session to reduce the cavity of the cyst.

According to the Gharbi classification, PAIR can be applied for stage 1 and 2 diseases, whereas care should be taken for stage 3 diseases not to remain any vesicles inside. For stages 4 and 5, it is not expected for the cyst to collapse and close itself, because of the calcification and the irregularity of the wall [11]. In such cases, if surgical intervention has been performed, at least one of the cavity-minimizing and secretion-reducing procedures such as omentoplasty, capitonnage, and intraflexion must be added to the procedure after the removal of the germinative and laminar membranes.

First, Khuroo et al. [12] compared percutaneous drainage of hepatic hydatid cysts with surgery and reported that percutaneous drainage with albendazole was an effective alternative to cystectomy. They found that percutaneous drainage showed similar efficacy in the regression and loss of cysts with the advantages of shorter hospital stay and low complication rate.

Zerem and Jusufovic treated 72 patients with univesicular and multivesicular hepatic hydatid cysts with percutaneous drainage by imaging with albendazole, and 81% of the cysts in the univesicular group and 63% of the multivesicular group were cured.

As a derived technique, Schipper et al. reported in 2002 that percutaneous evacuation of cyst content (PEVAC) is a safe and effective treatment for multivesicular echinococcal cysts with or without cystobiliary fistula, even though it is not used nowadays.

Hydatid cysts usually communicate with the biliary tree, which is a contraindication to the injection of sclerosing agents, as this may cause widespread injuries to the biliary epithelium [3].

7. Surgical procedures

The main purpose of surgical treatment in liver hydatid cyst is to eliminate the parasite, to prevent recurrence of the disease, and to minimize the complication and mortality by removing the germinative and laminar membranes. If the germinative membrane stays, asexual reproduction occurs, which is currently the actual recurrence reason of the cysts. Even if there are no vesicles left, sterile cysts may occur in the main location [13].

The main question here is: Is it necessary to remove the entire cyst, or is it sufficient to remove only the cyst? Two treatment modalities have therefore been proposed: radical and conservative surgery. The choice of surgical treatment depends on the number, localization, diameter, and complexity of the hydatid cysts, as well as the age and comorbidities of the patient, and the experience of the surgeon.

7.1 Surgical treatment indications

1. In large-scale uncomplicated CE2 and CE3b cysts with a large number of female vesicles [14].

2. In uncomplicated large cysts compressing adjacent vital organs.

3. In cases where percutaneous treatment is not possible.

    a. In spite of the possibility of spontaneous or traumatic rupture in superficially located and large single cysts.

    b. Infected cysts.

4. An alternative to percutaneous treatment in cysts with cystobiliary relationship.

7.2 Conservative surgical procedures

The basic principles of conservative surgical treatment are to clean all the contents inside the cyst and sterilize the cavity and to excise the pericyst as much as possible. Conservative surgical procedures are more simple and easier to perform than radical procedures. It is possible to perform these procedures in daily general surgical practice (**Figure 5**).

In conservative surgery, the basic principle is to open the cyst and sterilize the interior and then to manage the cavity. Various scolicidal agents are preferred for emptying the cyst content and for sterilizing the cavity interior. NaCl,

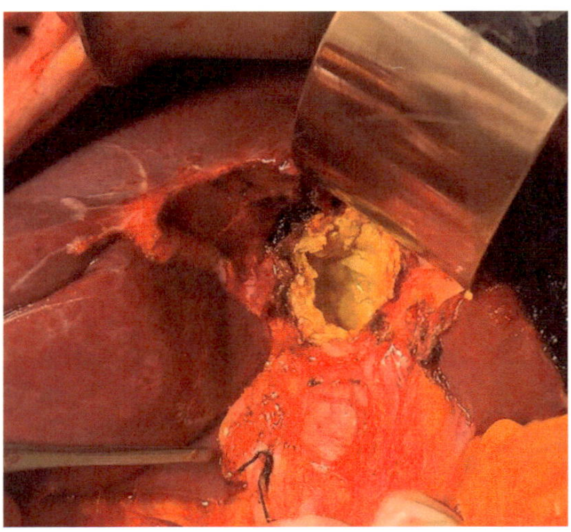

Figure 5.
An example of biliary duct connection of the cyst shown during the operation. A photo from our collection.

chlorhexidine, povidone iodine, ethyl alcohol, and hydrogen peroxide are used as scolicidal agents. The administration time of these agents is 5–15 min. Hypertonic NaCl and cetrimide are the most commonly used agents [15]. Different concentrations have been reported for hypertonic NaCl. Both clinical and experimental studies suggest that the scolicidal efficacy of a concentration below 10% is not sufficient. The ideal concentration is 20%. Each scolicidal agent must be prevented from contact with the bile duct, because they all have the potential to cause caustic sclerosing cholangitis. After emptying of the cavity, bile control should be performed. Bile leakage can be seen directly with the eye, or some researchers recommend to wash the cystic duct or choledochus with isotonic NaCl for detection of the bile duct invasion. It is recommended that all detectable bile ducts be carefully closed without damaging the common bile ducts. In cysts with large bile duct openings, caution is needed when using scolicidal agents and closing the fistula openings.

The second main part of cavity management is how to reduce or close the cavity. The cyst wall outside the liver parenchyma should be excised as much as possible, which is defined as partial cystectomy. After the cyst cavity has been minimized, the methods for the remaining cavity are unroofing, marsupialization, tube drainage, Posadas surgery and modifications (Llobet-Varsi modification), Roux-En-Y cystojejunostomy, and omentoplasty [16]. In the marsupialization technique, the edges of the cyst are sutured to the abdominal wall, and the cyst contents are drained out, which is now a historical approach. The technique that has been adapted to current surgical approaches is tube drainage, in which the cyst cavity is drained out of the tube, but postoperative complications are high. Posadas surgery and its modifications are used in small peripheral cysts with no biliary involvement and closure of the cyst after opening and emptying.

The current techniques used in the treatment of liver hydatid cysts are changing from simply unroofing the cyst to hepatic resections; the important part is to define the techniques. The cystectomy is basically opening the dome of the cyst and removing the germinative membranes and vesicles, whereas in pericystectomy, radical surgery is done by resection of the cyst with some liver tissue surrounding. Unroofing stands for the excision of the part of the cyst located outside the liver. Apart from the germinative membrane, parts of the cyst within the liver parenchyma are not touched when unroofing is done. The placement of a visceral organ, usually the omentum, into the cavity after unroofing is done is defined as quilting technique, whereas marsupialization is a historical technique in which building a tract from the cyst to the skin like an ostomy is done.

Although the most common indications for transduodenal sphincteroplasty are related to bile duct stones and cholangitis, this technique can also be used in hydatid cyst residues and membranes extracted from the common bile duct. The procedure may extend to the left and right hepatic channels, and angled Randall forceps are useful for this purpose. Sphincteroplasty involves suturing both sides or edges of the surgical sphincterotomy to prevent future stenosis of the incision. The sutures provide hemostasis in the incision margins and lead to the risk of retroduodenal perforation but also help prevent leakage of the duodenal content if it extends beyond the common portion of the incision line and sphincter.

Recent studies have reported postoperative morbidity and mortality rates of conservative techniques as 3–24% and 0–4% [17]. Although conservative surgical treatments are safer than radical procedures, they have become controversial due to the complications occurring in the postoperative period and the length of hospitalization. The most common complications are biliary fistula and cavity infection. Apart from these complications, bile peritonitis, cholangitis, and rarely sepsis and anaphylaxis can be observed in the preoperative period. Although anaphylaxis is extremely rare, it can be fatal. Hypernatremia is another complication that should be kept in mind in patients using hypertonic NaCl for cavity sterilization.

Although bile fistula is affected by various factors, it is observed in approximately 30–50% of cases. It is the most disturbing complication of conservative surgical treatment for the surgeon. The most predictive factor for postoperative bile fistula was found out to be the diameter of the cyst. Postoperative bile fistula rate increases in patients with a cyst diameter greater than 10 cm. Studies on the number, localization, and stage of the cysts on postoperative complications have yielded variable results, but localized cysts in the dome were definitely reported as a predictive factor. Postoperative bile fistula is defined as permanent bile fistula if it lasts more than 10 days. Endoscopic procedures are recommended primarily for the treatment of biliary fistulas. The cystobiliary fistula can be seen by ERCP, and endoscopic sphincterotomy, stenting, or nasobiliary drainage can be performed for therapeutic purposes.

An important problem during conservative surgery is the cavity infection. The rate of cavity infection in different series has been reported to be between 5.5 and 37%. Omentoplasty is thought to be useful in preventing cavity infection.

Mortality after conservative surgery can be seen up to 1.5%. Although higher mortality can be seen in patients with biliary involvement of the cyst, local recurrence rate is relatively higher in conservative methods than radical methods. Recurrences are reported to be caused by cysts growing from the pericyst to the liver parenchyma (exogenous vesiculation).

7.3 Radical surgical procedures

There are two radical procedures: pericystectomy and hepatectomy. In radical surgery, all the cysts can be performed with either excising the pericyst (pericystectomy—total cystectomy) or excising the parenchyma with the pericyst (hepatectomy) without opening the cyst. The rate of pericystectomy in radical surgery procedures is close to 90%. Unlike conservative procedures, radical procedures are more complex and difficult.

The pericystectomy is the preferred radical procedure because it is aimed to protect the healthy parenchyma as much as possible. There is a good dissection plan between liver tissue and cyst. Determining and progressing this plan will provide a comfortable dissection plan. When pericystectomy is performed laparoscopically, the operation is completed without emptying the cyst contents, and when the open method is performed, the pericyst is excised after the cyst is opened and the contents are emptied. Open method should be preferred especially in deeply located cysts adjacent to the hepatic artery or portal vein.

Indications for hepatectomy include the presence of large cysts that fill a lobe, multiple cysts, complicated cysts, and, according to some authors, being proximal to hilar vascular structures. This is an indication for hepatectomy if the large biliary tract is eroded. Particularly, lesions close to the inferior vena cava have been reported to be a partial contraindication. Caution is specifically needed for lesions adjacent to the right atrium and hepatic veins, especially the lesions in segments 1, 4, and 8. The radical resection is recommended for patients under age 75 only if the lesion is located with less than three segments of liver; if the residual liver function is sufficient to allow the surgery; if the vena cava, portal vein, hepatic artery, or biliary tract are suitable for repair; and if distant metastases are suitable for resection or do not cause life-threatening complications at least.

Complications vary according to the surgical method used in radical surgery. In general, complications related to liver surgery are observed and vary between 3 and 30% postoperatively. This rate is lower than conservative surgery. The advantage of radical surgery is that there is no cavity infection and the risk of biliary fistula is less (0.7–7%). The rate of infection in the surgical site is less than 3% in patients who underwent radical surgery. The low postoperative morbidity reduces the length of hospital stay in patients who underwent radical surgery. In addition, the possibility of local recurrence is less in radical surgery. The rate of local recurrence in conservative methods has been reported to be 20–25% in the literature, while the recurrence rate after radical surgery is 0.6–4%.

7.4 Surgical treatment of complicated cysts

It should be done according to complication. Biliary tract problems should be solved primarily in cysts that are involved with bile ducts. For this, ERCP and endoscopic sphincterotomy can be performed. Conservative methods should be used rather than radical surgery in free ruptured cysts to the peritoneum.

7.5 Minimal invasive surgery

The role of laparoscopy in the surgical treatment of liver hydatid cysts has always been discussed. The first studies were reported in the 1990s. The general advantages of laparoscopy, such as less hospital stay, less wound problems, and less pain, apply here. However, it is difficult to reach cysts in some localizations, and there are difficulties in aspiration of cyst contents and concerns about spreading of content and question marks about laparoscopy.

Reaching the cysts in the posterior and superior segments of the liver poses some technical difficulties. However, access to cysts in segments II, III, IVB, V, and VI is more convenient [16]. This situation also provides patient selection in liver hydatid cyst. In other words, laparoscopic or minimally invasive surgical treatment seems more reasonable for patients with cysts in the anterior segments. It can even be interpreted that laparoscopy is a relative contraindication for cysts in segments I and VII.

In addition, the cyst content is completely evacuated, and the possibility of spreading around while being evacuated is another problem. After the cavity is emptied and sterilized, it is aimed to perform cavity management with the same methods as in open cases [14]. After the cyst has been evacuated, laparoscopy can be used to magnify the bile leakage and suture the sources of leakage.

In laparoscopic surgery, exposure is usually caused by inaccessibility of the cyst, calcifications, and other complications (bleeding, etc.). The conversion rate to open radical techniques was reported as 1.7% [16]. At present, there is no obstacle to the treatment of liver hydatid cysts with minimally invasive surgery. In the published series, the recurrence rate in patients undergoing minimally invasive surgery is not higher than in open-operated patients. However, the indications of laparoscopy should not be forced, and patients should be selected well. As minimal invasive hepatectomies become widespread, minimally invasive radical surgery for liver hydatid cyst will increase.

8. Postop follow-up

Albendazole starting at 10 mg/kg/day should start to be used immediately for 6 months postoperatively. Hemogram and blood biochemistry should be performed every month (due to the risk of the toxicity of liver and bone marrow). Serological tests are not used in the early stages of follow-up (first few months), because none of them becomes negative in the early period. A control serological test (usually *Echinococcus* IHA) should be performed at the end of the 6-month postoperative period.

In this first 6 months postoperatively, USG is the main follow-up method. It shows both early recurrences and complications related to surgery. In the first few months, USG may show fluid accumulation in the cyst, which is usually seroma and will disappear afterwards. In recurrences, the fluid seen in the cavity in the previous USG will gradually increase.

Recurrence rates after surgery or invasive procedures range from 0 to 15%. The most common cause of recurrence is the scattering of living scolexes into the peritoneal cavity. Even if the patients is going to get operated, albendazole treatment is started 4–6 weeks preoperatively, which significantly reduces the risk of recurrence. The treatment of recurrent cysts is designed as in newly diagnosed cysts.

9. Alveolar cysts (*E. alveolaris* = *E. multilocularis*)

It forms 2–3% of liver cysts. In radiological imaging techniques, it is seen as the cyst wall makes papillary extensions into the liver parenchyma, which may resemble a hepatic tumor that leaks clinically and radiographically with irregular edges and heterogeneous density [18]. This formation is very important because if a part of the liver parenchyma is not resected in the surgery, there may remain a part of the germinative membrane which will cause recurrences (**Figure 6**).

There is also a PNM staging for alveolar echinococcal disease. P in the PNM shows the state of the parasite in the liver, N shows adjacent organ involvement, and M is for metastasis. Accordingly, PNM staging is as follows:

P: Shows the localization of the metacestode in the liver.

PX: Parasitic lesion cannot be evaluated.

P0: No parasitic lesion in the liver.

P1: Peripherally located and without biliary or proximal vascular involvement.

P2: Central lesion involving the biliary or proximal vascular structures in a single lobe.

P3: Central lesion involving the biliary or proximal vascular structures of two lobes, or involving two hepatic veins, or both.

P4: Any lesion extending along the portal vein, inferior vena cava, or hepatic artery.

N: Shows extrahepatic involvement to neighboring organs.

Nx: Unable to evaluate.

N0: No regional involvement.

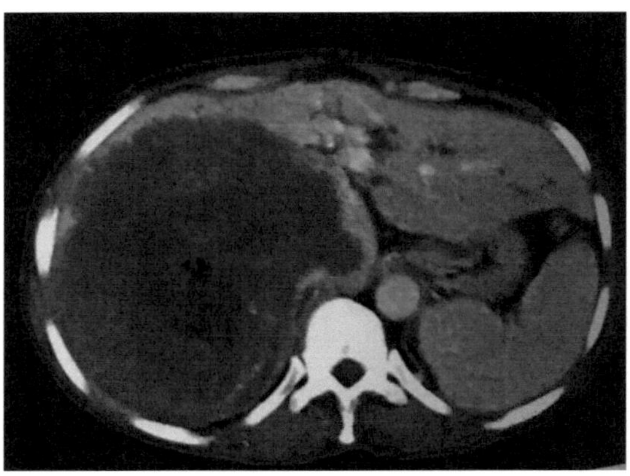

Figure 6.
Alveolar Echinococcus *lesion in right liver lobe shown in abdominal CT scan. Partial calcifications are seen around the lesion and left lobe is hypertrophied. Differential diagnosis with hemangioma is done with biopsy [3].*

N1: Involvement of neighboring organs or tissues.

M: The situation of metastasis.

M0: No metastasis.

M1: Metastasis.

The only treatment of alveolar hydatid cyst is surgery. Interventional radiological methods are not recommended. The surgical treatment should be pericystectomy, in which intact liver tissue of at least 1 cm should be excised with cyst. Within all operated hydatid cyst cases in Turkey, the ratio of alveolar echinococcus is about 15-25%.

MR and MRCP, and ERCP if necessary, are used preoperatively in each case considered for surgical treatment. Since pericystectomy will be performed, it should be known whether there is an invasion to the bile ducts, portal vein, or inferior vena cava.

Albendazole is used in cases where surgical treatment cannot be applied and in the postoperative period as well (as in case of all hydatid cysts). However, their daily dose should be higher, and the duration of use has to be much longer (at least 1 year).

In conclusion, alveolar hydatid cyst is a more resistant type and requires more aggressive surgery and medical treatment.

Conflict of interest

The authors declare no conflict of interest.

Author details

Mehmet Mihmanli*, Mert Tanal, Emre Bozkurt and Onur Guven
Department of General Surgery, Sisli Hamidiye Etfal Research and Training Hospital, Health Sciences University, Istanbul, Turkey

*Address all correspondence to: mmihmanli@yahoo.com

References

[1] Sahier M, Yalor MC, Greenberg HM. Canadian acquired hydatid disease: A case report. Canadian Journal of Infectious Diseases. 2001;**12**(3):178-182

[2] World Health Organization. Surveillance and Response, 2001 Classification. Department of Communicable Disease. WHO; 2001

[3] Belghiti et al. Sabiston's The Biological Basis of Modern Surgical Practice. 20th ed. Elsevier; 2016. pp. 42-48

[4] De Diego CJ, Olaverri FJ, Franquet CT, Zubieta OS. Computed tomography in hepatic echinococcosis. American Journal of Roentgenology. 1982;**139**(4):699-702

[5] Dryzska H, Sanghavi B, Peddamatham K. Hepatic hydatid disease: Findings on endoscopic retrograde cholangiography. Gastrointestinal Endoscopy. 1983;**29**(3):248-249

[6] Ul-Bari S, Hussain A, Malik A, Dass TA. Role of albendazole in the management of hydatid cyst. Saudi Journal of Gastroenterology. 2011;**17**(5):343-347

[7] World Health Organization. Tracking Universal Health Coverage. World Health Organization; 2015. ISBN: 978921564977

[8] Akhan O, Ozmen MN, Dincer A, Sayek I, Gocmen A. Liver hydatid disease: Long-term results of percutaneous treatment. Radiology. 1996:259-264

[9] Bret PM, Fond A, Bretagnolle M, Valette PJ, Thiesse P, Lambert R, et al. Percutaneous aspiration and drainage of hydatid cysts in the liver. Radiology. 1988;**168**(3):617-620

[10] Pedrosa I, Saiz A, Arrazola J, Ferreiros J, Pedrosa CS. Hydatid disease: Radiologic and pathologic features and complications. Radiographics. 2000;**20**(3):795

[11] Kelly K, Weber SM. Cystic disease of the liver and the bile ducts. Journal of Gastrointestinal Surgery. 2014;**18**:627-634

[12] Khuroo MS, Wani NA, Javid G, Khan BA, Yattoo GN, Shah AH, et al. Percutaneous drainage compared with surgery for hepatic hydatid cysts. New England Journal of Medicine. 1997;**337**(13):881-887

[13] Nunnari G, Pinzone MR, Gruttadauria S, et al. Hepatic echinococcosis: Clinical and therapeutic aspects. World Journal of Gastroenterology. 2012;**18**:1448-1458

[14] Schwartz's Principles of Surgery. 10th ed. McGraw-Hill Education; 2015. pp. 1052-1056

[15] Dziri C, Haouet K, Fingerhut A, et al. Management of cystic echinococcosis complications and dissemination: Where is the evidence? World Journal of Surgery. 2009;**33**:1266-1273

[16] Bostanci O, Kartal K, Yazici P, Karabay O, Battal M, Mihmanli M. Laparoscopic versus open surgery for hydatid disease of the liver. A single center experience. Annali Italiani di Chirurgia. 2016;**87**:237-241

[17] Tamarozzi F, Vuitton L, Brunetti E, et al. Non-surgical and non-chemical attempts to treat echinococcosis: Do they work? Parasite. 2014;**21**:75

[18] Engler A, Rong S, Beer M, Schmidberger J, Greater T. Simple liver cysts and cystoid lesions in hepatic alveolar echinococcosis: A retrospective cohort study with Hounsfield analysis. Parasite. 2019:26-54